INJURIES
IN
COMBAT SPORTS

By
Dr. GREG McLATCHIE

OFFOX PRESS OXFORD
1982

British Library Cataloguing in Publication Data
McLatchie, Greg
  Injuries in combat sports.
  1. Hand-to-hand fighting—Accidents and injuries
  I. Title
  617'.1027   RC1220.H/

  ISBN 0–9506989–2–X

Typeset by Oxford Publishing Services, Oxford
Printed in Great Britain by Billing and Sons Ltd.,
London, Guildford, Oxford and Worcester

DEDICATION

This book is dedicated to all who aim to maintain their health through sport and particularly to combatants who demonstrate singular fitness and courage.

Acknowledgements

I wish to thank all my friends and colleagues who have helped me produce this book. In particular Sam Galbraith, Paul Baines, Ian Steele, Jim Caullay, and Jim Mulligan deserve special mention. If the text has special merit it is due to advice and criticism from them as well as from Mr J S F Hutchison. Any faults in the text are my own.

For illustrations and support I am grateful for the generosity of the George Outram Company of newspapers, Mr K Davis, Smith and Nephew Ltd, Dr Charles McEwan, Mr J Caullay and Mr W Baxter of Bellahouston Sports Centre, and Napp Laboratories.

Neither the author nor the publisher can accept any liability for any injury resulting from the reader's interpretation and application of the advice given.

PREFACE

Combat sports always have been and always will be with us.
In recent years various campaigns have been launched to ban or
outlaw certain of them for either medical or ethical reasons. The
fact that combat sports have become so popular, and that so
many people of their own free will want to take part in them,
makes the prospect of banning them almost non-existent. The
need is therefore to find ways to help the people involved by
teaching them how to recognise and deal with the many injuries
and problems they will be facing, and more importantly by
teaching them that a great many of the problems can be avoided.
Dr Greg McLatchie's book could not have come at a better time.
In his career he has managed to combine a doctor's knowledge
with an athlete's experience, and he has found a way to pass on
both of these accomplishments in a language that everyone can
understand. Athletes push their bodies beyond all limits and
therefore they expect to have aches, pains and injuries. Combat
sportsmen, because of the nature of their sport, probably have a
much lesser regard for pain than other athletes and so they tend to
"live with" or "train through" injuries that really should be
given proper treatment.

In many cases the only medical advice available to an injured
athlete is that of his G.P., who will no doubt insist that the injury
be given complete rest. Unfortunately, for an athlete training
towards a deadline, complete rest is usually out of the question,
and he must find a way to keep working while the injury is being
treated. In this situation Dr McLatchie's book will be of
tremendous help because he is not looking at the problem purely
from a medical point of view but is also looking for a practical
solution. It is really surprising that athletes who rely so heavily
on their bodies can go through a whole career without taking the
trouble to learn even the simplest things about how their bodies
work. I am confident that this book will go a long way towards
making all sport much safer and much more enjoyable for those
taking part. My only regret is that the book was not available
when I was setting off on my own career.

JIM WATT
World Lightweight Boxing Champion, 1979–81

FOREWORD

Take two of these pills if the pain gets too much, and have two weeks off.—The only way to get better is to rest.—It's a strained muscle here. Have a week off.—The only thing you can do with a back injury is lie on it for a few weeks and rest.

In all my twenty-six years of judo, seventeen of which were in the British team, I must have heard that type of advice hundreds of times, both from hospital doctors and General Practitioners. Doctors often do not understand the difference between the normal sedentary person and the sportsman, particularly the international competitor. When I go to my doctor I want positive and constructive help and advice, both about the rehabilittion of an injury and, more importantly, about the prevention of such injuries in the future.

I am what you might call a full-time sportsman who works to a very strict training programme, which leads to a competition—it may be the British, European or World Championships. It could even be the Olympic Games, which is the pinnacle of a lifetime of training. No sportsman wants to hear negative comments on injuries and problems which occur during normal training and competitive life.

Coaches, Managers, helpers, trainers, doctors and physiotherapists only advise on the rehabilitation of the injury. They don't advise on prevention.

This book covers all aspects of the sports injury scene—psychological, sociological, injury management, legal problems, fitness, strength training in rehabilitation after injury, and diet. It is nice to read positive advice from a doctor when you know that you must do some training to keep in condition for that big competition. Everything is covered in the book, from small injuries to major problems. Most important of all is the author's entry into a new field—that of prevention. I can speak from experience: it is true that prevention is better than cure.

This book is a must for all who have an interest in sports, from Mums and Dads to doctors.

BRIAN JACKS
European Judo Champion 1964, 1965, 1970, 1973
and Olympic Bronze Medalist 1972

CONTENTS

PART II INJURY MANAGEMENT

9. ABOUT INJURIES 70

1.
THE MANAGEMENT OF INJURY IN COMBAT SPORTS

In the last ten years the number of people who participate in regular sport has increased enormously. The Sports Council has estimated that approximately fifteen million people take part in regular sports activities in Britain today and the Government actively encourages sporting endeavour through its 'Fit for Life' campaign. Sport then provides an effective, satisfying means of spending our increasing leisure time and nurtures a feeling of physical and mental well-being for millions. Participation promotes health and improves the quality of our lives.

One of the most rapidly growing sports of the last decade is, perhaps surprisingly, combat sport. This broad term encompasses many diverse activities ranging from boxing to kendo, from wrestling to full-contact karate. Although dissimilar, the basis in history of all these sports was attack or defence in life-threatening situations. They have since evolved into 'sports' and often bear little resemblance today to their original forms.

Although boxing itself has diminished in popularity since the war, other combat sports have largely filled the gap it has left. Especially popular are the oriental martial arts which increased in popularity during the seventies through the media of cinema and television. These facts, linked to an increase in municipal violence, have encouraged many people to acquire a practical fitness applicable also in the form of self-defence.

However we view the benefits of sporting activities of any kind, there can be little doubt that the only deleterious effect of 'Sport for All' is injury. As doctors interested in the prevention and treatment of injuries in sport we feel that this aspect of the sporting boom has been considerably understated. Many people take part without being aware of either potential hazards or of how to treat injuries. This is most important in relation to combat sports where misapplied or ignorantly directed techniques can result in death or disablement. Most injuries can be prevented if you learn to recognise the situation in which they might arise.

There are many combat sports practised in Britain today. We have divided them into three separate types:

1. Those which are predominantly punching or kicking (or both): Boxing, Thai Boxing, Karate, Full Contact, Hapkido, Nihon Kempo, Kong Soo Do, Kuk Sool, Kung Fu, Tai Chi Chuan, Tang Soo Do, Tae Kwon Do.
2. Those which are predominantly grappling or throwing (or both). These also involve the study of the articulation (and disarticulation by locks!) of joints: Judo, Aikido, Wrestling, Jiu-Jitsu, Hapkido.
3. Those which predominantly involve the use of weaponry: Kendo, Kobudo, Hwarang Do, Nin Jitsu, Escrima, Kyudo.

We have adopted this classification not because of any necessarily similar philosophical aspects, but because the injuries which occur in each group of sports are similar.

We would emphasise, however, that any type of injury can occur in any of the sports, from a simple bruise to a brain injury. As the coach, instructor or participant you should be aware of the range and risk of injury in your particular activity.

TAKING CONTROL OF INJURIES

The key to success in any combat sport is control. The fighters must be able to control their aggression so that they don't flail wildly at each other. The referee must be able to control the fight and the governing body must be able to control the sport. It may seem to many of you that there is sometimes too much control. However, one area where there is still perhaps too little control is in the prevention and treatment of injuries.

This book has been written to allow coaches, trainers, participants and the governing bodies to take greater control of this part of the sport and to give them information which will help them make safe and wise decisions. Too many injuries occur which could have been prevented and too many injuries are incorrectly treated. Our purpose then is to help prevent and treat injuries. The book does not, of course, remove the need for a doctor, physiotherapist or chiropodist. We have tried to indicate when such skills are required and when an injury can be managed by the coach or fighter without professional help. We believe it will give coaches the feeling of being in greater control when injuries occur and when fighters ask how injuries can be prevented and how to prevent recurrent injuries. We hope you will become fascinated by this preventive aspect of injury management and that you will try to increase your knowledge by attending first-aid courses and the officially organised courses run by the governing bodies of some combat sports.

We shall discuss many types of injuries, but all can be considered as one of two kinds, depending upon their cause. There are those which result from overuse and those which result from trauma (direct or indirect violent forces). Overuse injuries are often gradual in onset and unrelated to blows or twisting. They are difficult to diagnose and treat and should be left to the doctor or physiotherapist in most cases.

Those which result from trauma are usually of acute onset, being caused by a punch, kick or some sudden body movement. We hope that this book will give you basic guidelines on the assessment and management of these traumatic injuries.

THE CRUCIAL DECISIONS

Timing

Timing is always important in combat sports. The fighter with good timing is set apart from his fellows. He knows just when to slip and counter, when to take an opening, or when and how to create a scoring chance. Timing is equally important in the management of injuries and in the course of each injury there are three times when crucial decisions have to be made.

1. Is the injured person fit to keep fighting? This is the first important decision.
2. Does he need a professional second opinion? This is the second important decision. It may have to be made in the ring or on the mat or even in the dressing-room. Sometimes the problem may not arise until weeks later when an injury which originally appeared minor is not recovering as expected.
3. Is he fit to restart training? This is sometimes the most difficult decision.

Urgency

All injuries should be treated as quickly, but as calmly, as possible. However, when it has been decided that a second opinion is required from a doctor, it is not always necessary to obtain it quickly. Some cases require medical attention more urgently than others and throughout the book we use the same three terms for the three degrees of urgency.

As soon as possible

When we say medical help should be sought as soon as possible, that means *immediately*. The player should be taken to hospital. If you take him, ensure that he is given *nothing to eat or drink* in case he needs a general anaesthetic.

The same day

When this phrase is used the problem is less urgent. The fighter should call his general practitioner, but if he is unavailable or unwilling to see him, the fighter will have to go to hospital. With this type of problem the fighter may return to his home town before seeking treatment if the injury is sustained when he is playing in an away match.

Make an appointment to see a doctor

Some injuries should be seen by a doctor but do not need to be seen the same day that the injury occurs. For such injuries it is sufficient for the person to make an appointment with his doctor even though he may have to wait several days before the doctor can see him.

HOW TO USE THIS BOOK

If you buy a power-drill or motor mower you will be given a set of instructions. We would hope that this book will become as useful to you at competitions and in the dojo as a power-drill or motor mower is at home.

The chapters of this book are arranged in two parts. The first, and more important, part describes the ways in which the risks of injury can be reduced and injuries can be prevented. It is impossible to over-emphasise the importance of injury prevention or the part that coaches and trainers have to play in prevention. You will often need the help of highly-trained professionals to treat the injuries that will occur from time to time, but highly-trained professionals — doctors, dentists and physiotherapists — can only treat injuries: they cannot prevent them. Coaches, trainers, officials and referees are those who have the opportunity to practise preventive medicine. The social importance and legal implications are also described because above all the combat sportsman is a member of society and must not abuse his skills. In recent years there have been reports by senior police officers that they have noted an increase in 'martial arts'-type postures in people who have resisted arrest or have been involved in fighting. Forensic reports have also been brought forward on the use of half-learned martial arts skills to knock a victim out before further assaulting him.

The second part of the book deals more directly with injuries. After a general introduction to the principles of injury management and a chapter on handling emergencies, a series of chapters cover the different parts of the body. In each chapter in this section the anatomy is described, and advice on injury prevention is given, followed by a brief description of the common injuries, with the signs that indicate the need for expert help emphasised. Finally the way in which the fighter can be helped to regain fitness to train and fight is discussed.

Many injuries produced in combat sports are unintentional and occur because the 'attacker' has been unaware either of basic human anatomy or of the injury process. We have therefore tried to cover these important aspects early in the second part of the book, underlining the need for understanding injuries and preventive measures before describing particular injuries and their treatment.

We would like you to read the whole book, from start to finish, so that you get a feeling for the whole subject. Try to discuss the points raised in the different chapters with other coaches and trainers and exchange ideas on injury prevention. Compare your first-aid bags and see what other people find useful. Then you can consult the book when you need it, but we hope that you won't simply use this book like a gardening book, leaving it on the shelf most of the time. Use it like a road atlas, take it with you in your pocket or bag. It is a textbook of 'touchline' medicine to be used at competititions or training sessions. Don't be ashamed to consult it on the dojo, at training or in the dressing-room after the fight. We do not expect you to carry all the information in your head when you can carry it in your pocket. One piece of advice is that we recommend you to consult the book openly. Involve the injured person and tell him you are going to check to see if he needs a doctor. Make him feel the confidence we hope you will gain from reading this book.

Finally, don't rely on the book alone. It won't make you an expert, although it will tell you how to make the most effective use of the expert help available. Enrol in a first-aid course run by either the British Red Cross Society, the St John Ambulance Association and Brigade, or the St Andrew's Ambulance Association. In this book we have not tried to teach you how to do mouth-to-mouth resuscitation because we believe that it is not possible to do this by words alone. You need a practical demonstration and the opportunity to try the technique using the apparatus which the first-aid courses organised by these associations use. We believe everyone should attend a first-aid course not just because it complements the knowledge about the management of combat sports injuries which we hope you will acquire from this book, but because it includes teaching on other problems, for example burns and scalds, which we believe everyone should know about. These organisations may also be able to help you by the provision of trained first-aiders if you are organising a big tournament. Contact one of the organisations and find out when you can enrol in a course.

The three organisations have jointly produced an excellent book called *First Aid* which can be purchased at any branch or in any major bookshop. It is well worth reading but is best read while attending a first-aid course.

These first-aid courses do not cover every topic — it would be impossible for them to do so in the time available and you will benefit from further instructions even if you have already attended a first-aid course. Try to find enough support among your colleagues in your own and other clubs to make it worth-while for your local association to mount a course on the prevention and treatment of injuries in combat sports. Find a physiotherapist or doctor who works near you who is inter-ested in sports medicine and ask if he would organise one, or more, teaching sessions for coaches and trainers.

Remember also that you can learn a great deal from other coaches and trainers, for example:

What is the best way of preventing abrasions?

What equipment for the treatment of injury should be

available in the club?

What should be carried in the first-aid bag?

What type of clothing is the most effective for the prevention of injury?

What should be done to control a fighter who seems to enjoy injuring his opponents?

These are the types of question that the experienced coach can answer as well as the most highly-trained professional.

THE GOLDEN RULES

Stay safe

In a competition or boxing match it is sometimes necessary to take risks in order to break an opponent's defence. This may be all very well if the fighter has made the decision himself, but when you are involved in managing the injuries of other people there is no scope for taking risks. Therefore if you are responsible for a decision affecting the well-being of another person, you have to be much more cautious than if you were making the same decision about yourself. As you will read later, combat sport involves specific injuries which can be dangerous both in the short and the long term. Your decision-making should be especially careful when it applies to youths and children. There will be occasions when you must refuse absolutely to let a fighter take a risk by either entering a match after an injury or by continuing to take punishment even though he says he is coping.

Remember too that your decisions regarding young fighters and children in combat sport may have legal as well as medical implications. These are discussed at length later. Do not be too afraid of the legal implications. If you have acted in a reasonable and sensible manner no court would hold you responsible, but as the coach or trainer you must be especially aware of the possible effects of even an apparently mild injury. A knowledge of risk situation is also expected of you.

Just as you have to be more cautious with others than you would be with yourself, we have had to be more cautious in the advice we have given than we might be if we were standing beside you at the ringside or mat. We have followed our own rule — *Stay safe*.

Stay cool

Keeping cool under pressure is a requirement for any good fighter. His coach must stay cool too. Don't shout angrily and uselessly at fighters, whether your own or the opposition. A cool, confident approach prevents panic and allows constructive thinking. The coolness and economy of movement of the great boxer Joe Louis at his peak reflected the efficiency of his training. If you sustain an injury (or your fighters get injured) you must also stay cool. No matter how anxious you feel, try not to show it or you may sustain further injuries. If you are the coach you may make your fighter anxious.

As the coach you must reassure the injured fighter. Put a blanket or towel round his shoulders. Smile reassuringly and look confident. Research has shown that the pain people feel after injury depends both on the extent of the injury and also, surprisingly, on the confidence they have in those around them.

Finally, never fool yourself. Don't become too confident, but let your outward appearance be calm and reassuring — *Stay cool*.

Look and listen before you touch

When someone gets injured do not rush in and grab the injured part to examine it. Look at the injury, talk to the injured person. Ask him where it hurts, can he bear weight, can he remember what happened, and so on. Is there an obvious deformity? Compare the injured part of the body with the same part on the other side of the fighter. Look at and feel the uninjured hand, knee or ankle so that you learn a little bit about the player's normal anatomy. Only after all this should you consider touching the injured part — *Look and listen before you touch*.

Prevention is better than cure

Always think prevention in combat sport. It is a difficult concept to promote since it is in no way so dramatic as gushing blood or broken bones. It is, however, extremely important. When an injury occurs ask yourself 'How could this have been prevented?' Use the knowledge for the future.

We shall discuss prevention later in the book but start your reading with this motto in mind — *Prevention is better than cure!*

2.
RISK FACTORS IN SPORT

'The only exercise I took was to attend the
funerals of friends who took exercise.'
Mark Twain

Although few people would adopt the cynical attitude of Mark
Twain it is true that almost all forms of sport involve risk. This
is what adventure is about and is one reason why we all enjoy it
so much. However, we believe that you should make a logical
decision about the risks involved. What must be decided is
whether the risks of a particular activity are acceptable or
whether they can be minimised without damaging our enjoyment to any great extent. Such a decision demands that you are
aware of both risks and gains.

PERSPECTIVE

In this chapter we shall put sports into perspective with respect
to injury and compare combat sports with others. We hope also
that you will begin to identify risk factors in your own sport
and think of ways to prevent injuries.

Look at the figures listing the frequency of injury in various
sports. You will note that the 'high injury' sports are rugby
football and soccer. Boxing and judo rank well down the list.
However, competition karate has an injury rate which is even
higher than that of football. It is apparent from Fig. 2 that a
football injury which is significant enough to be reported will
cause about a week's lay-off. However, a boxing or judo injury
regularly produces a very long lay-off time — up to six weeks.
This is because many injuries in combat involve the head or a
major joint. These are potentially more serious than a simple
bruise and require a longer time to recovery.

These findings are not surprising if we consider that the
original intention of combat was to disable an opponent. This
risk is still present in the sport. It is therefore in your own

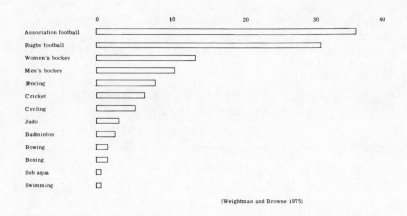

Fig. 1 Number of injuries per 10,000 man hours of play for each sport (13 selected sports).

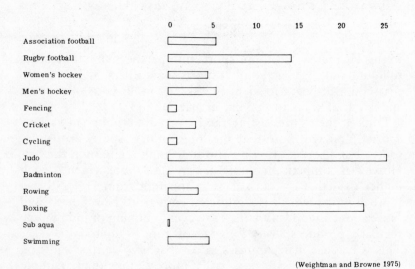

Fig. 2 Median days off play per injury per season.

interest to avoid injury, for more than likely it will stop you participating for weeks or perhaps even several months.

There are several sports other than combat where the risks used to be high but have been reduced by clever use of preventive measures, without spoiling the game. These are worthy of further detail.

Rugby football

There has recently been tremendous interest in the subject of neck injuries in rugby football. These can cause permanent paralysis. At an international match during Wales' centenary year several former rugby players were invited as guests. They sat in their wheelchairs on the touchline! All had sustained broken necks playing rugby.

It is now known that the risk of a neck injury is increased by scrummaging on a wet pitch and by collapsing the scrum. The Rugby Union has wisely instructed referees to penalise players guilty of this manoeuvre. It may take a few years before we see a changing trend in neck injuries but the decision would seem to be a sensible one.

In another study on rugby a group of doctors noted that almost one third of all injuries resulted directly from foul play. The implication of this finding is that injuries could be reduced considerably if foul play was eradicated. But violence in sport is such an accepted form of cheating that it will take some time before this risk factor is removed. In this study only one-tenth of all fouls were penalised. Fouling an opponent is breaking the rules. If this occurs in a combat sport the outcome may be very serious indeed. We would encourage each governing body to issue firm policies concerning foul play which leave neither the participants nor the referee in any doubt as to what action will be taken.

A further study in a contact sport — football this time — showed that in one season one fifth of the players in the ten teams studied sustained some sort of dental injury. In following seasons this sample group was recommended to wear mouth shields and there was a subsequent reduction in injury.

Cricket

Other sports have changed too. In the 1960s who would have

thought we would see cricketers wearing crash helmets and visors to prevent injury? Yet even in this increasingly competitive 'gentleman's ' game it became apparent that certain types of bowling could be effectively pitched short of the batsman so that the ball would ricochet at head height. This was a part of the 'psyching-out process' used by bowlers. It was also very dangerous indeed — a result of the extreme desire to win. Padding, gloves, helmets and visors are now the rule — and all this in a game where the intention is basically to hit a ball with a bat and score some runs as a result!

These examples are given because they emphasise the scope for intervention by the governing body in injury prevention. Sensible interpretation of injury statistics enhances the safety of players. We are aware of the enormous contribution made by the boxing associations to the medical care of the boxer. Could greater safety measures be taken? In the other combat sports are there injury situations which you recognise? If so, you should encourage discussion with your colleagues, the club physiotherapist or doctor and your governing body. Awareness leads to safety.

DISPELLING MYTHS

It is incorrect to interpret literally the old fighting motto 'No pain, no gain', for when applied to injuries it will almost certainly be 'Pain, no gain'. Most injuries in sports are to the soft tissues — the skin, muscles, tendons and ligaments — of the body. Although damage to these may appear trivial in comparison to broken bones, they can produce persistent pain and discomfort, eventually becoming a 'weak spot'.

The object of all training is to acquire physical fitness and skill. Ideally, it should not produce injury. How can you give total commitment to a competition if you are anxious about the painful knuckle that you hurt two weeks ago in training? Remember that the clever fighter is skilful because he avoids injury during roadwork and sparring. He trains sensibly and safely.

PREVENTION OF INJURY

Look backwards to look forwards

Prevention in medicine is nothing new. None of us would willingly drink water into which unprocessed sewage drained. Why? We know we would become ill with dysentery or cholera. Yet the young doctor who first suggested that contaminated water supplies in London were the cause of so much ill-health and disease found an enormous political struggle on his hands in his efforts to get his idea accepted and educate people in this preventive aspect of health care.

Last century another young doctor reduced the rate of infection in maternity wards almost overnight by simply washing his hands between examinations! Until his innovation childbed fever was an extremely common cause of maternal death. For his observations he was forced by jealous colleagues to leave the country. So preventive measures do not always increase popularity.

The enormous advances in health care (not treatment) this century have been due in the main to effective preventive medicine. Killer infectious diseases such as smallpox, tuberculosis and poliomyelitis have all but been eradicated. Now public attention is directed towards the prevention of 'social disease' related to cigarette smoking or heavy drinking. Perhaps in the twenty-first century the answers to these problems will also be obvious in retrospect.

So be encouraged that preventive measures are usually simple. Count the number of injuries occurring in your club in a year. Does wearing protection in sparring or fighting reduce the number? Learn to identify risk factors and carefully avoid them, both for your own protection and for that of your colleagues.

How teamwork helps to prevent injuries

Each person in your sport or associated with it is a member of a team which comprises:
1. The instructor or coach
2. The participants
3. Referees, seconds, judges
4. The club doctor and physiotherapist
5. The governing body

Each team member should be aware of the common injuries and how to prevent them. It follows that this would also allow more time to be devoted to treatment of those injuries which remain. We should all learn to identify injury situations and to control them. Participants should adhere to the rules. Referees should be able to make fair decisions based on the policies of the governing body which supports the referee's decision. The medical team, which may involve a doctor, nurse, physiotherapist or trained first-aider, should not only be able to offer assistance when injuries occur, but also to give information on injury statistics and to offer advice on injury prevention. Regular meetings with all concerned in combat sport would do much to achieve this end.

INJURY SITUATIONS

In all the martial arts there are three areas of participation where injury can occur. They are:
1. Non-contact practice on one's own
2. Striking objects
3. Non-contact pre-arranged sparring, free sparring and competition.

Solitary practice

This can include the warm-up with flexibility exercises and kata. These can also be performed in groups. Most problems in this category are caused by injudicious or over-enthusiastic warm-up. Instructors should not push pupils past the limits of their flexibility by methods such as jumping on the knees during seated adductor muscle stretching or pushing on the back when stretching the hamstrings. Another frequent cause of adductor injury is doing forced splits either fore and aft or sideways. The best method is to allow the pupil to set his own limits. If exercises are performed to the onset of discomfort and the position reached held for ten to fifteen seconds, much quicker progress will be made.

The injuries most prevalent in this group are strains and sprains, yet few are reported. Students continue practising and in so doing exacerbate a quite treatable acute injury which subsequently becomes a chronic problem.

Striking objects

This includes the use of punch bags, punch balls, makiwara, sandbags and also tameshiwara (breaking objects). Training is generally performed with the bare hands and feet.

The commonest sites of injury are therefore the hands and feet, with nerve injury to the hand and fractures of bones in both hands and feet presenting a major risk.

Protective changes are also known to develop, such as thickening of the skin over the little finger border of the hands and callouses on the knuckles. These can produce considerable discomfort and may even become infected.

Prearranged sparring, free sparring, competition

Similar injuries result from these three groups. Only in pre-arranged matches is there more control since each partner should know his/her role. In free sparring and competition there are many variables which promote the types of contact which cause injury.

Vague tournament rules and poor officiating

The control exerted by the referee is immediate. He is in charge of the fight. Remote control is exercised by the governing body in that it sets the rules and regulations. The referee interprets these. Experience is important for the referee. Competitions can be very heated with considerable crowd participation. It is vital that the referee sticks to his decisions even in such situations. The support of the governing body for the referee is obviously essential.

Cheating

Any infringement of the rules is cheating. We have already discussed the relevance of violence in sport with reference to rugby football. It is also possible for violence in combat to be regarded as cheating. If a fighter uses any illegal technique he infringes the rules. Furthermore, because of the nature of the sport, serious injury can result.

Another form of cheating is the use of too much bandaging on the hands of the punchers. The application of all bandages should be witnessed and only regulation lengths used.

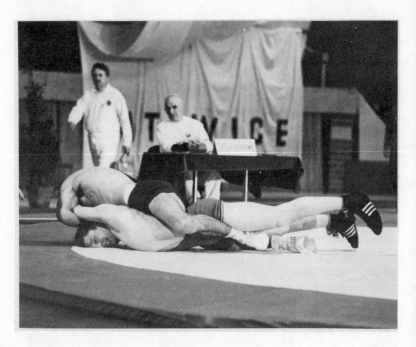

Fig. 3 Cheating. With his left heel firmly in his opponent's crotch in the first movement of a Polish Hank, extra leverage for the lock is obtained by applying the force against the opponent's elbow instead of his head as is usual.

Lack of protective clothing and equipment

The indoor training area should be well ventilated and illuminated. There should be adequate floor space to avoid collisions with other competitors. We recommend the use of sprung flooring for boxing rings and padded or matted flooring for other combat sports. These measures do prevent serious injuries.

Studies have confirmed that protective clothing also reduces the number of injuries. This can be a head guard in boxing or a body protector in contact karate. We advise you to wear such protection in sparring.

Differences in body weight

Depending on the sport no competitor should outweigh his opponent by more than seven to fourteen pounds.

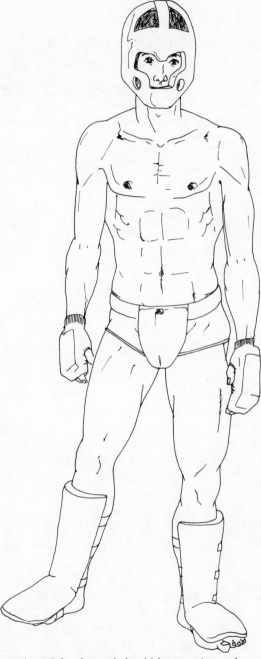

Fig. 4 Protection. A head guard should be prominent above and below the eye.

Inexperience

Most injuries will occur in inexperienced fighters. However, when an injury occurs in an experienced fighter it is generally more serious.

There are also situations where an experienced fighter will be sparring with a relative novice. The former must exercise great care, for the novice may not anticipate the attacks. His poorer reactions may lead to injury.

3.
THE SPORTS

'Wild animals never kill for sport. Man is the only one ...'
James A Froude

INTRODUCTION

Those sports which derived from original combat are of three types:
1. Predominantly punching like boxing and karate.
2. Predominantly grappling and throwing like aikido, judo, jiu-jitsu and wrestling.
3. Weaponry like kendo, fencing and use of weapons in karate.

Our reason for this division is that the injury situations which arise are similar in each group. Sites of injury tend also to conform to each group, although it must be remembered that an injury can occur to any part of the body from any sport.

PUNCHING ARTS: BOXING

At one time boxing was so popular that important world events such as the 'French revolution' were poorly reported on the back pages of newspapers because they clashed with an important fight. It remained so until the end of the Second World War since when boxing has given way to pursuit of other pastimes. There are now about 7,000 bouts per year in Britain.

In many ways boxing has been the most instructive of the combat sports in medical terms. When it was very popular it became apparent that regular fighters developed slurred speech and a swaying walk. This became known as being PUNCH DRUNK. It is caused, as you will read later, by sustaining many minor head injuries, the effects of which add up over the years. When this was recognised there was public criticism of boxing and attempts were made to ban it. The result was that now boxing is probably one of the best medically controlled sports, with considerable reduction in serious head injuries and still further attempts to make the sport safe.

A standard bout lasts for three to five rounds in amateur boxing and up to fifteen rounds in professional boxing. Standards of refereeing are generally high and medical recommendations are strictly enforced. These apply mainly to prevention of head injury.

However, early fights such as that between Epeus and Euryalus in 1100 BC were very different. For the prize of a mule the fighters clubbed and lacerated each other wearing gloves called CAESTI. These were leather gloves impregnated with spikes or iron or lead studs. Head protection was provided by leather helmets. The rules were that the victor should not kill his opponent. Epeus won by a knock-out.

Boxing continued to develop through the Roman circuses but after the fall of the Roman Empire references to the sport are scant. The first recorded British champion was in the late seventeenth century. Eye gouging was still legitimate in these contests which gave way to barefist fights with rules and then the modern sport.

The first boxing rules were drawn up in 1743. Compare them with those of today. You will see similarities.

Rules of boxing (1743)

In 1741 the English champion (Broughton) beat a contender who subsequently died. At first the champion swore he would not fight again, but relented provided that in future fights the following conditions were fulfilled:

I.   That a square of a yard be chalked on the stage and on every fresh set-to after a fall, or being parted from the rails, each Second is to bring his man to the side of the square and place him opposite to the other, and till they are fairly set-to at the lines, it shall not be lawful for one to strike at the other.

II.   That in order to prevent any Disputes, the time a Man lies after a fall, if the Second does not bring his Man to the side of the square within the space of half a minute, he shall be deemed a beaten Man.

III.   That in every main Battle, no person whatever shall be upon the Stage except the Principals and their Seconds: the same rule to be observed in bye-battles, except that in the latter Mr Broughton is allowed upon the Stage to keep decorum, and to assist Gentlemen in getting their places, provided always he does not interfere in the Battle; and whoever pretends to infringe these Rules to be turned immediately out of the house. Everybody is to quit the Stage as soon as the Champions are stripped, before the set-to.

IV.   That no Champion be deemed beaten unless he fails coming up to the line in the limited time, or that his own second declares him beaten. No Second is to be allowed to ask his man's Adversary any questions or advise him to give out.

V.   That in bye-battles, the winning man to have two thirds of the Money given, which shall be publicly divided upon the Stage, notwithstanding any private agreements to the contrary.

VI.   That to prevent Disputes, in every main Battle the Principals shall on coming on to the Stage, choose from among the gentlemen present two Umpires, who shall absolutely decide all Disputes that may arise about the Battle; and if the two Umpires cannot agree, the said Umpires to choose a third, who is to determine it.

VII.   That no person is to hit his Adversary when he is down, or seize him by the ham, the breeches, or any part below the waist; a man on his knees to be reckoned down.

These original rules governed prize fighting until 1838 and after several revisions were superseded by the Queensberry rules in 1866. Further revisions continued until the British Boxing Board of Control produced the current rules.

Particular injuries

The main target of attack (the head) and the instrument of attack (the hand) are the commonest sites of injury — indeed injury elsewhere is rare.

Head injuries

These are described in detail in Chapter 11. They are the commonest cause of death and serious disability in the sport. For this reason amateur boxing is usually restricted to three rounds. The ten- and fifteen-round contests are retained because of public demand.

Rules governing a knock-out. After knock-out the boxer is not permitted to fight for a four-week period. Both amateur and professionals will require a medical examination before re-entering the ring. In the case of the professional boxer a scan of the brain's activity is also required (electro-encephalograph). If an amateur boxer sustains more than three knock-outs in a year he is suspended indefinitely pending further medical examinations. In the case of a professional boxer who has had three knock-outs in a year the suspension period is three months. He also must be certified medically fit before returning to the ring.

Cuts, injuries to eye, ear, nose

The injury section deals specifically with these. You should refer to it for details.

Hand injuries

These are extremely common. More than half of all injuries will occur to the hand. Obviously it is important to do all that is necessary to avoid injury. A hand injury can keep you out of the ring for months.

The most frequent injury is fracture or fracture dislocation of the thumb, especially of the large joint at the base of the thumb. The main reason for this happening is the position of the hand in the glove (it sits in a separate compartment) and poor delivery when the blow is struck.

Other injuries which occur are broken (fractured) knuckle bones, especially the index and little finger knuckle.

Such injuries are painful, can take weeks to heal but most important they can be PREVENTED.

Prevention of Injury in Boxing

Head injuries

Head injuries can be prevented to some extent by always sparring with headgear on. Contrary to popular belief your brain does not get used to being knocked about. So wear headgear.

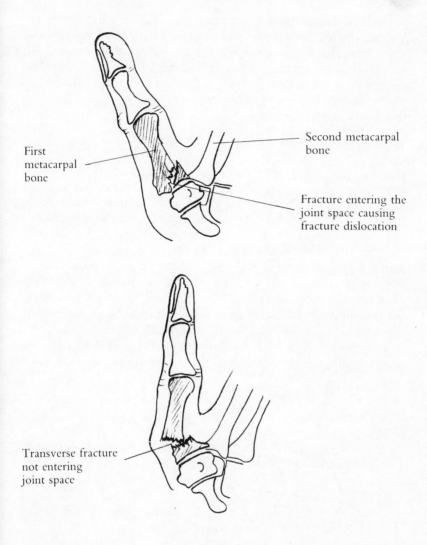

First
metacarpal
bone

Second metacarpal
bone

Fracture entering the
joint space causing
fracture dislocation

Transverse fracture
not entering
joint space

Fig. 5 Common injuries to the bones of the thumb in Combat Sports.

Do exercises to strengthen your neck muscles. Wear a gum
shield. Above all, if you are knocked out even momentarily in
training, stop sparring for that evening and train only on the
bag for the four week period afterwards. This will not be
popular advice but it goes a long way towards preventing
serious problems later.

In the fight situation the referee must know what to do. He should know about the effects of even minor head injuries and apply the rules to the letter. What is the point of allowing a man to continue when he is not in charge of his faculties? The referee's responsibility is to see a fair and safe fight, not satisfy the crowds. That is the fighter's responsibility and he achieves this by being fit and skilful.

Hand injuries

Hand injuries can be prevented by ensuring that correct punching techniques are taught. The coach should be able to demonstrate this. You should strike with the index and middle finger knuckles because they are immobile and the force of the blow passes directly to the solid arm bone — the radius. Make a fist yourself. Note how the knuckles of the ring and little finger move down as the fist tightens. Now grasp each knuckle of your hand in turn and try to move them up and down. This does not happen with the index and middle finger knuckles. When you practise punching, your fist should be in position so that the striking knuckles hit the target (Figure 6).

The glove design with the thumb in a different compartment makes injury to the thumb likely. More recent designs have

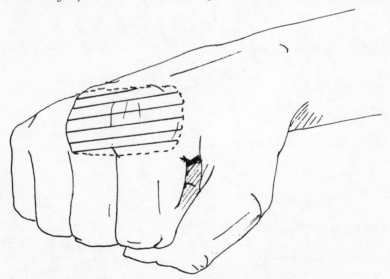

Fig. 6 The striking knuckles of the fist.

incorporated a flange so that a blow to the thumb will glance off it. However, you must still practise correct striking. Try to keep the thumb firmly applied to the rest of the glove when actually punching.

Gloves. The first gloves were introduced by Broughton in England in the mid-eighteenth century. Their purpose was to protect the face and hands in training. Later on gloves were used in championship fights. Until the early 1900s they were skin-tight.

Today six-ounce gloves are used in fights up to and including welter-weight, and eight-ounce gloves from middleweight on and in all amateur contests.

Further developments in the form of pneumatic gloves are currently under examination. For light sparring, ten- and twelve-ounce gloves are recommended.

Tapes. Bandages or tapes are permitted for *protection of the hands*. They must not exceed nine feet of one-inch zinc oxide plaster tape or eighteen feet of two-inch soft bandage for weights up to and including middleweights. Light-heavy and heavyweights are allowed eleven feet of zinc oxide plaster tape. If a fighter uses more than these lengths or applies tape over his knuckles he could seriously injure his opponent.

IT IS VITAL THAT THE REFEREE AND/OR DOCTOR CHECKS THE TAPE AND THAT AN OFFICIAL WIT-NESSES ITS APPLICATION. BOXING GLOVES SHOULD BE PUT ON IN THE RING SO THAT THE REFEREE CAN INSPECT THE TAPED HANDS.

PUNCHING ARTS: KARATE

Historical background

Karate, in modern Japanese, means 'empty hand' and in its simplest sense this implies empty-handed combat without the assistance of weapons. In its deepest sense it implies infinity of knowledge, self-discipline and religious conviction.

Although its origins can be traced to China, modern karate is said to owe its development to the Ryukui islanders who, when overrun by the Kyushu in 1609, cleverly circumvented the veto which banned weapons of any kind by devising an empty-handed form of combat so effective that a trained exponent could punch through the bamboo armour of his oppressors with his hardened fists, or dismount horsemen with high kicks. As practised today, it still has two distinct forms — the one a philosophical way of life linked strongly to the Zen religion; the other a practical martial art concerned with the acquisition of spectacular physical skills and historically linked to the ideology of Bushido (the way of the warrior), the code of conduct of the Samurai.

The concept of Bushido

Bushido was a highly specialised code of honour and conduct which the Samurai warriors of feudal Japan were required and instructed to observe. It loosely related to chivalry in that it dictated both how the fighting nobles should behave in battle and in their daily life. It was an unwritten code which had grown out of centuries of military life. For those who diligently adhered to its concept it meant absolute loyalty to their immediate superiors and thus unquestioning obedience. The Samurai had to be prepared to fight and die without the slightest hesitation, to be oblivious of pain and have no fear of death. Obviously they were daunting adversaries. The code stressed the necessity of not pondering the pros and cons of a superior's command, so that orders were carried out immediately, without deliberation. It also laid down minute rules of etiquette and methods of dealing with vanquished opponents who did not conform to the precepts of Bushido.

The concept of Bushido pervaded Japanese thinking. It applied to all aspects of life — especially during the Second World War — and also of course to the teaching and learning of martial arts.

The acceptance of pain as being a necessary part of advancement in Japanese karate is one reason why there was an initial high injury rate in the sport. This principle has gradually been eroded on common-sense grounds. Most people who practise karate in the West are not monks and have to work for a living. Injury causes valuable loss of time from work and, sometimes more important, sport.

Forces in karate

The most extraordinary feats in karate such as breaking wood or smashing concrete blocks are explicable scientifically. The 'secret' of the karate blow is the concentration of the body's energy in a small area on the target. By taking strobe pictures of punches and kicks the energy delivered can be calculated. In a straight punch forces of 675 lb/sq inch are generated by a good standard karateka (black belt and above). More force is required to break wood than concrete. This may seem surprising, but wood is more elastic than concrete and requires a lot of energy to deform it.

However, all karate exponents know that wood is easier to break than concrete. In the collision between hand and target only part of the energy is transferred to the target — the remainder is transferred to us and is known as pain! Wood will absorb most of the hand's kinetic energy, but concrete obstinately refuses at least half of it. This presents a psychological problem to even the most hardened karateka and exaggerates the difficulty of breaking concrete compared with wood.

Why don't the bones of the hand or foot break? Provided the force of collision is directed along the lines of stress in the bone no break will occur. Bone is tougher than wood or concrete but the striking hand or foot must be held in the correct posture. Remember this in all aspects of your practice.

Karate competitions

Most competitions are one of three types:
1. Traditional — controlled contact
2. Semi-contact
3. Full-contact

We have found that, by careful interpretation of the rules and the strict application of medical recommendations, injuries can be reduced in all types.

1. *Traditional*

A basic awareness of human anatomy would permit easier scoring of competitions. Since no actual contact is made in most karate competitions, arguments arise as to the efficacy of a punch or kick. Therefore we have included anatomical drawings in later chapters to assist you in making your own decisions. Perhaps this will stop arguments and reduce frustration in fighters who feel they have made a good point.

2. *Semi-contact*

Most injuries in competition occur to the limbs because of persistent low kicks. There are inherent dangers in kicking the legs and we would respectfully suggest a revision of the rules especially with regard to breaking boards between each round. This has produced many unnecessary injuries which cause loss of time from sport and work.

The application of a points system alone and less emphasis on the knock-down in this style of karate may permit improvements in injury statistics.

3. *Full-contact*

The lesson has been learned from boxing. The same rules must be applied in relation to knock-outs. Fighters should be well matched and of equivalent weights. Sparring should be conducted in protective gear.

Full-contact karate is now increasing in popularity and seems to be filling the gap left by boxing. There are many inherent dangers in this sport since the addition of the feet as weapons compounds the risk of serious injury (Fig. 7). There is a general awareness of this, however, and to date many fights have been well-controlled. The most significant injuries are to the head but also to the liver, kidneys and spleen. Other injuries such as sprains and strains do occur but are over-shadowed by the potential of more serious injury.

Preventive measures must be directed towards stringent rules: full pre-fight medical examination, strict refereeing by informed referees and the standard recommended lay-off times after injury.

Particular injuries

Head injuries

The potential for knock-outs always exists even in non-contact karate. Skull fractures can result from falling backwards and striking the head on a solid floor during sweeps or after an uncontrolled punch to the face. The full-contact sport presents

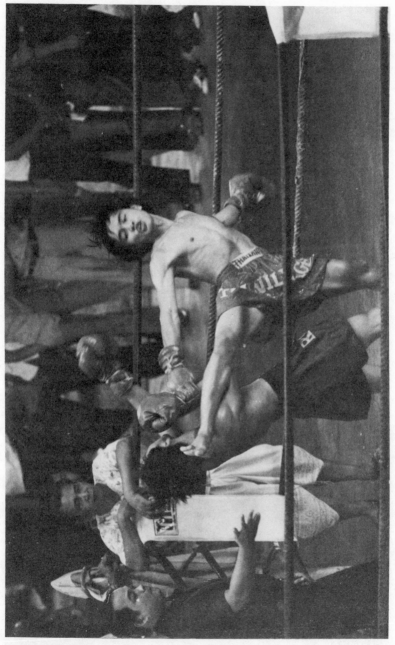

Fig. 7 In Thai boxing and Full Contact Karate the use of the feet compounds
the risk of injury.

exactly the same head injury problems as boxing and therefore stringent medical rules regarding fitness to fight should be implemented and all fights should have a doctor in attendance. For full details on head injuries read Chapter 11.

Trunk

The commonest injury is 'winding'. This results from a blow or blows in the region of the 'pit of the stomach' (where the rib cage meets the abdominal muscles near the midline). The injured person has extreme difficulty breathing in, due to transient paralysis of a large breathing muscle called the diaphragm. Fortunately the sensation usually passes off in about thirty seconds and no treatment other than sitting forward with knees bent is required. We have seen some referees chop the injured person on the back. THIS IS A VERY DANGEROUS PRACTICE AND SHOULD NEVER BE DONE.

If the person does not recover quickly, take him out of the fight and arrange for him to be transported to the nearest casualty department for examination. THIS SHOULD BE DONE PROMPTLY.

Testicles

The Japanese word is 'kintecki'. They are a recognised target on all self-defence body charts but are mostly accidental victims in contests. A blow here is sickeningly painful and can produce unconsciousness or vomiting at worst. Again the pain usually passes off quickly and most contestants continue to fight. After such an injury always inspect your penis and scrotum or get a responsible colleague to look. If there is bruising of the penis or scrotum GO TO HOSPITAL FOR EXAMINATION PROMPTLY.

If a person continues to have pain after a blow to the testicles ARRANGE FOR QUICK TRANSFER TO HOSPITAL.

MOST OF THE MARTIAL ARTS REFEREES WILL DIS-QUALIFY A MAN WHO IS NOT WEARING A GROIN GUARD IN COMPETITION. THIS MAY MEAN THAT YOUR OPPONENT COULD WIN IF THE REFEREE DEEMS HIS BLOW ACCIDENTAL — ROUGH JUSTICE INDEED!

Limbs

The hand, as in boxing, is one of the commonest sites of injury. The fingers can be dislocated from attempts to parry blows and toes from effectively blocked kicks. You should refer to the appropriate chapters to see how to deal with these.

Bruises and breaks can affect the main limb bones also (see injuries sections).

Nerve injuries

One particular group of injuries which do occur in karate are nerve injuries. The nerves most often affected are:

1. *The radial nerve* in the upper arm. A kick to the mid part of the upper arm can temporarily 'knock the nerve out'. The person complains of weakness of his grip and also of tingling over the arm and back of the hand. Such nerve injuries can sometimes be associated with a fracture of the humerus (upper arm bone) and may require surgical repair.

   Historically kicks (mawashi-geri) to the mid upper arm prevented an armed man from gripping or wielding his sword.

2. *The ulnar nerve* (funny bone). Most often injured from kicks to the elbow, the ulnar nerve injury produces tingling of the little and ring fingers and half of the hand and weakness of their muscles.

   Another site of injury of the ulnar nerve is in the hand. It supplies muscles on the chopping side of the hand and can be damaged if the student over-enthusiastically strikes firm objects over a prolonged period. One such unfortunate student presented to his doctor with wasting of all the muscles on the 'chopping' border of his hand due to swelling of this deep branch of the ulnar nerve. When he stopped doing tameshiwari his problem reversed. A salutory warning to all would-be wood breakers!

3. *The superficial peroneal nerve.* This nerve is most often injured during a sweep. The person complains of tingling and weakness of the foot. Symptoms usually settle in hours but may persist for several weeks. If the symptoms have not settled by the next day see your doctor.

Recommendations

Over the last seven years we have studied more than 7,500 karate contests of all styles and types. Our overriding conclusion is that the following factors will reduce injuries in combination by a factor of 5 to 10 depending on the type of karate. We strongly advise you to ensure that the folowing precautions are in force when you fight.

1. Protective padding to the shins, feet, arms and hands.
2. Gum-shields.
3. Equivalent body weights.
4. The use of padded or well-sprung flooring of the standards recommended by the Martial Arts Commission. This recommends padding of at least 1 cm thick as floor covering. It should ideally be of the interlocking type.
5. Reduction in importance of wood breaking.
6. Medical cover at competitions.

Many arguments have been mooted against these recommendations but all studies performed confirm that a combination of the above factors reduce both the number of injuries and their severity when they do occur.

EVERY PERSON WHO TEACHES KARATE SHOULD HAVE ALREADY ACQUIRED BASIC FIRST-AID KNOWLEDGE BY JOINING THE RED CROSS, ST JOHN'S OR ST ANDREW'S FIRST-AID CLASSES. (See Chapter 10.)

GRAPPLING AND THROWING ARTS

Judo

In the mid 1860s, a Japanese college professor, Dr Jigaro Kano, began a detailed study of the many ancient fighting forms of the Orient. He realised that each fighting school saw their concept as superior to all others. After many years of study he synthesised all he had learned and called the art judo — the gentle way. He argued that the most efficient way of fighting was to use intellect, personal ability and your opponent's mistakes. Thus, if he threw a punch you could throw him using his own momentum.

Judo is now an extremely popular sport for young and old people. It is very popular amongst children and is a recognised Olympic sport in which Britain has consistently performed well over several Games.

Judo involves rapidly changing one's centre of gravity to perform throws and the use of groundwork and locks to maintain an opponent in a helpless position. Locks against the joints and the application of strangles or chokes are characteristic of groundwork. In experienced hands the lock or choke can be applied as a throw is completed so that the opponent is held firmly on the mat — a scoring position.

Aikido

This Japanese martial art was originated by the Morihei Ueshiba and subsequently adapted and modified into various schools, second-generation modifications of which have appeared in Britain.

The sport involves redirection of an attacker's energy with grappling and striking. It also involves some use of weapons.

Approximately 1,300 persons practice the art in Britain.

Jiu-jitsu

This Japanese martial art is of uncertain origin and great antiquity. It involves throws, locks and holds with ancillary strikes to weaken or divert the attention of an opponent whilst a grappling technique is applied with the object of gaining a submission. Self-defence against weapon attack is also taught.

The art developed in several areas independently and therefore several schools of style persist today. The Martial Arts Commission has estimated that there are around 2,250 practitioners in Britain.

Particular injuries

Strangles and chokes can cut off the blood and oxygen supply to the brain and produce unconsciousness. You will read later that these episodes of unconsciousness can add up in their effect to produce permanent brain damage. So all episodes of unconsciousness after strangles should be treated subsequently in a similar manner to head injuries. These latter can result directly from poorly performed breakfalls or accidents with the various types of weaponry which may be used in demonstrations.

The most commonly injured joints are the shoulders, elbows and fingers. Mat burns, grazes and bruises are common. Fortunately, serious abdominal injuries are rare.

Injury situations — prevention of injury

Most injuries happen when:
1. A breakfall is poorly executed (Fig. 8).
2. A limb lock is over-enthusiastically applied or not submitted to (Fig. 9).
3. A choke or strangle is applied too long.

The wrist, elbow and head are the injury sites after poor breakfalls. Effective prevention lies in adequate warm-up and frequent falling practice. If an injury to a major joint (wrist, elbow, shoulder, hip, knee) does occur, the affected limb should be supported gently, either with broad bandages lightly applied, or on pillows or sandbags, until professional assistance is available. Do not attempt any heroic reductions of such dislocations in the dojo. The techniques can be effectively learned by attending professionally organised first-aid classes.

As a competitor it is important that you are able to draw the line between accepting excessive pain and simply being stupid. As a referee, you must continue to watch carefully any limb lock or strangle and should be encouraged to decide early whether or not a fighter has sustained enough punishment.

Wrestling

Wrestling is not exclusively an oriental-based combat sport. It is one of the oldest sports in the world and probably the most widespread. By 3000 BC in Egypt it was already a highly-organised scientific sport with complicated rules and protocol as is witnessed by over 4,000 holds and throws inscribed on the walls of the tombs at Ben-Y-Hassam.

Many reports abound of famous fights: Ulysses and Ajax wrestled at funeral games before the walls of Troy; Rusterm killed Sohrab, his son, before the King of Afghanistan — even today the Indian champion is called Rustern Hind; in the 14th century, when Turkish tribes made raids into Europe, two men

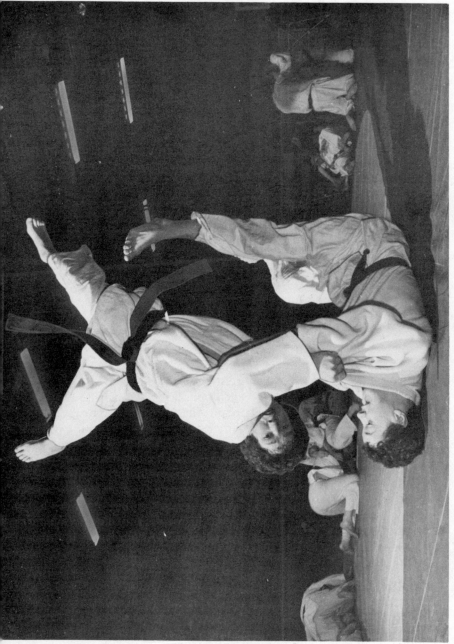

Fig. 8 A judo throw. If the breakfall goes wrong, the wrist, elbow and shoulder can be injured.

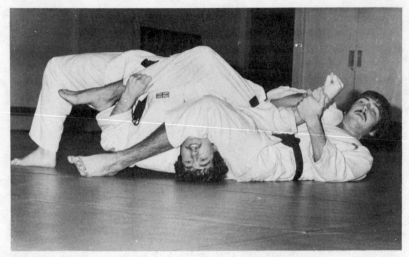

Fig. 9 Arm locks also put joints at risk of dislocation.

wrestled for three days without decision, then died of exhaustion. As a result a three-day wrestling tournament has been held each year on the site ever since.

To unite these disparate international traditions the modern Olympic style of wrestling developed. It is a standardised form of the traditional styles and contains their inherent strengths and diversities. This is the reason for its world-wide appeal.

Even today many cultures measure courage by wrestling ability and several Eastern countries send only wrestling teams to the Olympic Games. Indeed in Turkic languages the word for hero and wrestler is the same — 'Pehlivan'.

In Britain three types of wrestling are practised:
1. Olympic or free-style
2. Graeco-Roman
3. Professional

Fighters must have well-cut nails, short hair, and be of equivalent weight. No jewellery is allowed in fights. In free-style wrestling any fair hold is allowed. In Graeco-Roman wrestling holds below the waist are forbidden and trips or throws using the legs are also illegal.

All-in professional wrestling is a spectactular sport where no holds are barred — save direct chokes — and the forearm and flat of the hand are permitted as instruments of attack. Although apparently extremely violent, injury and death are very rare. In the last forty years only two deaths have occurred — one due to a heart attack, the second to head injuries after falling out of the ring.

Professional wrestling would seem to provide a high degree of safety for the wrestlers and crowd satisfaction — especially for female fans!

Particular injuries

The most serious injury in wrestling is cervical dislocation. Because the wrestler's neck is hyperextended during a bridging manoeuvre, the injury tends to be at a high level, sometimes simulating a hangman's fracture (see neck injuries, Chapter 15). It is essential that only legitimate methods be used to break the bridge. Sudden pressure on the arch of the bridge (chest and abdomen) will almost certainly produce cervical injury.

Another common group of injuries is those to joints, especially the knee and shoulder. Many of these can become chronic and disabling. Treatment at the time of injury is recommended.

Grazes, facial cuts and mat burns are extremely common. Of these mat burns can be very painful and if wrestling continues the burned area should be carefully covered to protect it. The initial treatment of burns is described elsewhere (Chapter 9). Grazes and facial cuts usually respond to simple first-aid measures. If extensive, expert help may be required.

Injury situations — prevention of injury

Neck strength is essential. All trainee wrestlers must begin by practising gentle bridging exercises. As expertise increases, kick-over bridging and bridging with weights can be practised (Fig. 10). During the souplesse or salto techniques some wrestlers land on their foreheads in the bridged position. This demands immense muscular strength and timing. Such a forehead landing should not be attempted by novices. It may be better for them to 'rotate-out' so that their full weight and that of their opponent does not stress the cervical vertebrae.

Neck-strengthening exercises are also an important part of injury prevention. Effective strengthening can be achieved by using weights in the shoulder-shrugging and pulling exercises,

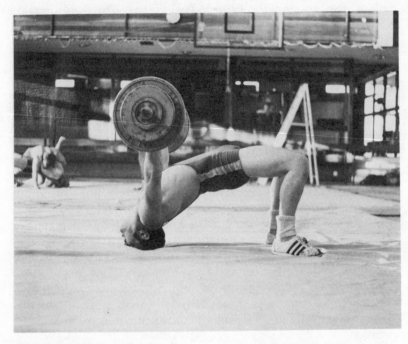

Fig. 10 Neck strengthening exercises reduce the risk of injury. This wrestler demonstrates exceptional strength.

keeping the weight as vertical as possible and close to the body.

Contestants should have short hair so that there is no impairment of vision. Pre-fight medical examination and rest periods after head injury or nasal bleeding are mandatory. The doctor present must decide whether a man can continue after injury.

No hold is allowed which will cause a man to submit because of pain. No strangleholds or holds against a joint's normal movement are permitted (free style and Graeco-Roman).

WEAPONRY

Fencing and kendo are variations of combat sports in which the original sword is substituted with an epee or shiai respectively. Both sports have long histories but, since they make the use of protective equipment mandatory serious injury is rare and does not require further detailed discussion. The commonest

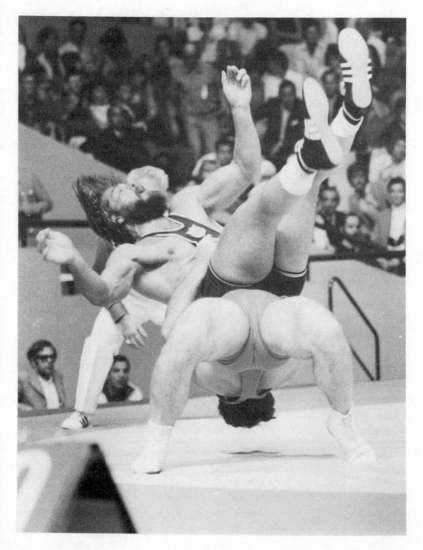

Fig. 11 Should you land on your forehead in a full bridge or twist off just before impact? In the Souplesse technique it is important to have extremely strong neck muscles.

problem encountered is bruising, usually to the chest and upper arms. These are rarely troublesome in the long term.

There have been two reports of death resulting from kendo

accidents. The mechanism is worth noting, for it underlines the importance of ensuring that protective equipment, if worn, is *in good condition*, and also emphasises that frequent inspection and care of weapons is essential for preventing injury. In both cases death was secondary to eye injuries. The shiai shattered. Bamboo splinters penetrated the face guard and the eye socket. One victim of such an accident died from a blood clot on the brain, the other from infection. Only last month (July 1982) the tragic death of a top Russian international fencer was announced. His death resulted from a penetrating orbital injury after his opponent's foil had broken. Once such an injury occurs, infection can set in, making treatment very difficult. At all levels of sport where weaponry is involved prevention is a most important aspect of training. These injuries are avoidable.

More common causes of death in weapon sports result from non-symptomatic heart disease and older competitors have died naturally from heart disease while fencing.

Use of weapons in karate

One extension of karate is the use of oriental farm implements as weapons. We encourage extreme caution when teaching the use of such apparatus. Strict control of the class and slow, repetitive movements are necessary before mastery, demonstrated by blinding speed and co-ordination, is achieved. The inexperienced may find their weapon more injurious to themselves than to any imaginary opponent.

4.
SOCIETY, THE LAW AND COMBAT SPORTS

> 'We live in a freakish world, a vicious world.
> People like to see blood.'
>
> *Mohammed Ali*

SOCIETY AND COMBAT SPORTS

All societies have enjoyed combat sports. In ancient Rome the gladiatorial 'games' involved the spectacle of men or women fighting each other or animals to the death. It was entertainment for the spectators. Somehow they would manage to distance themselves from the carnage they witnessed to enjoy the contest. If a gladiator fought well, the crowd would signal to the director of the games that he should be set free. Poor fighters were not so fortunate. Their lives rested on the whim of the crowds and were frequently terminated. Litter would be thrown at the victim as the 'execution' took place.

In October 1980 a frail-looking diabetic, Johnny Owen, was beaten unconscious. As he lay being counted out the Tequila-soaked spectators threw plastic cups full of urine into the ring. Johnny Owen died several weeks later from serious head injuries. Little has changed since the days of the gladiatorial games. It seems that we sublimate our aggression through fight heroes. They are our champions who represent whatever ideal or emotion we wish. In the excitement of combat it is very easy to will injury on the opposition without necessarily wishing permanent damage to be inflicted.

The death of Johnny Owen and of several other boxers throughout the world revived public interest in the sport. Private bills were presented in an attempt to ban boxing, but these failed. Earlier, in the sixties, Lady Summerskill had begun a crusade against boxing. Although unsuccessful, she prompted the Royal College of Physicians to carry out one of the most detailed medical studies ever performed on former boxers. The results showed that one fifth (20%) of former boxers suffered some degree of brain damage. Detachment of the retina with subsequent blindness was also relatively common. Death in the ring occurred four to six times per year. These findings were published in the early sixties.

The boxing authorities took the message seriously. So effective was their medical control, especially in the amateur sport, that no case of brain damage has been reported since 1974. Eye injuries still present a problem however, and the death of a fit young man is a tragedy which still occurs occasionally.

What are the alternatives? The sport, and the newer combat sports, could be banned. This would almost certainly drive them underground, increasing risk. We feel that if combat is to remain a safety valve for our aggressive society, the injury team described in Chapter 2 must work harder at eliminating risk factors in order to make the sport safer.

How can this be done and the people still have their 'bread and circuses' as in Rome? We must change our philosophy towards injury. Instead of being seen as part of the game injury should become almost unacceptable. And is it always necessary to injure someone to win? Stricter refereeing, increased medical cover, examination of fighters in all combat sports and the use of protective equipment — perhaps even in the fights — would do much to improve the situation. The fight spectacle would still exist — the injuries might not.

SOCIAL VIOLENCE AND SELF-DEFENCE

It is now generally believed that we live in one of the most violent periods of human history. Riots are commonplace and the number of individual assaults has increased. A new word — 'mugging' (= kicking, assaulting) — has been introduced into our everyday language and police figures confirm that this is the most common method of homicide after stabbing and strangulation. Against such a background it is not surprising that combat sports are so popular. They offer self-defence and physical fitness *par excellence*. Unfortunately, perhaps, guidelines are required and demanded even for the innocent party of an assault.

Use of skills outside the combat arena

There are legal implications to possessing self-defence skills. If you find yourself in a dangerous situation outside the ring or dojo you may be forced to *defend yourself*. It is important that, in the eyes of the law, you use only the minimum force necessary to get yourself or someone else out of the dangerous situation. This is now a real fight — no referee to control foul blows or judge to give you points for artistry. You may also be terrified — this is quite unlike your sparring or competition situation. The use of violence by you will only be condoned by the law if you:

i)   are protecting yourself
ii) are protecting other people

and only if there is extreme danger and no other means of escape or retreat. Your retaliation must only be the minimum necessary to protect your own or someone else's life so that you can make a getaway. The measure of retaliation is not exactly specified and the court would make allowance for fear or excitement. However, a complete 'non-fighter' in such a situation *might well be allowed a much greater degree of error* in his assessment of *the effect of a blow* than you would with your knowledge of combat sport.

Assault? — The concept of 'game' versus 'fight'

When you take part in any sport you imply that you will abide by the rules and also imply your consent to accepting any reasonable risks that exist. What happens when these rules are broken? If a rugby player retaliates by hitting his opposite number, is this just high spirits? There is no difference in law between this and punching someone in the street. The two are equally assaults and both criminal. The only difference is that in the sporting context there will probably be no formal complaint lodged about the assault and hence no criminal proceedings; in the public context a complaint is likely to be made, resulting in criminal proceedings. Remember, however, that where sporting assaults are brought to the attention of the authorities they are dealt with quite severely, and further, such incidents may give rise to civil remedies for damages. In the last few years we have noted several convictions against sportsmen for violent behaviour on the field of play. You cannot consent to being assaulted.

Obviously in a combat sport the interpretation of what constitutes an assault is wide. However the following could be interpreted as assault:

i) An illegal punch in boxing, such as a rabbit punch to the back of the neck.

ii) In controlled-contact karate, deliberate lack of control producing injury to another person could constitute an actionable assault.

iii) Any illegal kick or throw in full-contact karate, traditional karate or judo.

Our advice is that you should know the rules of your sport and stick to them firmly. Do not be tempted to cheat. Someone may be seriously injured and you may end up with a conviction for assault.

'Tadpole' and 'Toad'

To help illustrate the foregoing principles the tale of 'Tadpole' and his aggressive acquaintance 'Toad' may prove useful.

1. 'Tadpole' is aged 16 years and very slightly built for his age. He has, however, been attending karate classes for three or four years, has done quite well in competition, but has never been involved in any 'real-life' fights.

2. 'Toad' is an extremely well-built 19-year-old who is quite well known in the area, and is certainly known to Tadpole, as a weight-lifter of some considerable note.

3. Toad is at a disco and is slightly (but not very) drunk, and for some reason, apparently quite unjustifiably, takes a dislike to Tadpole.

4. Outside Toad hurls verbal abuse at Tadpole, who quite sensibly (in view of his size in relation to Toad) simply does not reply and makes to clear off.

5. This seems to annoy Toad, who runs up behind Tadpole and pinions his arms. In law, at this point, Toad has inflicted a *criminal assault* on Tadpole.

6. Because of Toad's strength, his action is extremely painful for Tadpole, who quite cleverly screams loudly and causes Toad to release his hold to try to silence him. Tadpole, managing to divert Toad's attention momentarily by stamping on his foot, runs off. In law Tadpole has not been guilty of an assault in stamping on Toad's foot. He has not in any way used excessive force, and he has done the right thing in running away.

7. Tadpole runs up an alley to get to another street, but because of a gas pipe being up, there is a high temporary hoarding blocking off the alley. Toad quickly catches up with Tadpole.

8. Tadpole is in a state of considerable fear and alarm, for he is now cornered. Remember he has never been in a fight before in spite of his karate skills, and Toad is extremely powerful.

9. Toad, even further annoyed at Tadpole, and still slightly inebriated, advances towards Tadpole, whom he does not in any way rate as an opponent because he is so small. Probably because of that he simply strolls leisurely up to Tadpole.

10. Tadpole, however, has realised that he is going to be assaulted, and has decided to endeavour to use his skills to protect himself. Completely to Toad's surprise, Tadpole lands a very severe blow to his leg, which causes Toad to fall to the ground in considerable pain.

11. This leaves the way clear for Tadpole to escape, but surprised and really rather pleased at himself, he does not do so.

12. Toad is trying to get up, still in pain, and now more concerned with his leg than with Tadpole. The inevitable onlookers have arrived.

13. Tadpole, now flushed with his success, and no doubt spurred on by an audience, proceeds to land further blows on Toad, who, much to the onlookers' astonishment (and no doubt Toad's) is completely unable to defend himself. He is, within a very short time, senseless.

14. Tadpole leaves the scene. Toad is fortunately not seriously injured. He is bruised about the body and, more seriously for his weight-lifting, has a dislodged knee-cap.

15. Analysing the position in law we would point out that Tadpole did not commit any actionable assault the first time he struck Toad, as it happens on the leg. He did not, in the circumstances, use unnecessary force, but it was that blow that did the serious damage, and which, had it not been justified, could well have given rise to a civil damages claim because of the potential long-term effects on Toad's weight-lifting. Thereafter, however, Tadpole could and should have made his escape. The blows he subsequently inflicted were undoubtedly criminal assaults on Toad, even though Toad had been the original aggressor, and while Tadpole could have pleaded PROVOCATION in mitigation, each blow he struck would make that less and less relevant.

16. In the event, although the police became involved, Toad prevailed upon them not to pursue charges, no doubt because

he was the instigator of the incident and also probably because his pride was considerably hurt.

However, if you use more than the minimum force necessary to defend yourself you may not be so fortunate.

Legislation for control of combat sports

National legislation involves a complex process whereby a law is passed and enforced. This is unlikely to happen in sport. Internal legislative control is therefore exercised by the governing bodies with co-operation from clubs and associations. It is a process of good will and social responsibility. The main governing bodies of each combat sport are recognised by, and lists of them are obtainable from, the Sports Council.

Combat sports can be extremely dangerous to both participants and public. They should only be taught by qualified persons to suitable students.

There is therefore a need to control teaching and practice of combat sport by:
1. Ensuring that teachers are adequately qualified.
2. 'Screening' participants and maintaining a control register (as in professional boxing).
3. Allowing facilities for training to be available only to competent instructors.
4. Ensuring adequate medical back-up.

We strongly encourage you to become a member of a Sports Council recognised body. This will ensure both your safety and an acceptable standard of expertise. At present, most people practising combat sports will be members of the Amateur Boxing Association (ABA), the British Judo Association (BJA), the Martial Arts Commission (MAC) or the British Wrestling Association (BWA).

Responsibility

Many clubs give training contracts which have to be signed by the club members. These contracts usually carry indemnity clauses which state that the club cannot be held responsible if a participant is killed or seriously injured whilst practising a combat sport (this applies especially to martial arts clubs). They are only effective if all reasonable precautions have been taken by the club to ensure safety. This applies to contests too. The safety regulations are well described in these pages. Your club is responsible for ensuring that reasonably safe premises are in use.

Each participant must also be responsible for and to him/herself. If you honestly feel that there is a danger area at your club it should be reported to the instructor. This is fair to yourself and others.

A further aspect of this relates to the treatment of injuries. Each club should have a well-equipped first-aid box, but more importantly there should be a member, trainer or instructor who is competent in its use present at each training session.

These measures ensure safety but also increase the confidence of both instructor and student.

Children in Combat

Children under the age of sixteen are not regarded as being responsible to make decisions regarding their own safety. A child, therefore, cannot join a club of his own free will. The parents should give signed consent after the implications of the training have been explained to them. At all times children should be carefully supervised and should certainly not be expected to perform feats of strength such as wood breaking, press-ups off their knuckles or hardening techniques for the hands. This can produce damage to growing bones which may be permanent. The club may also find itself legally obliged to compensate for such injuries.

FORENSIC MEDICAL ASPECTS OF COMBAT

Accidental death?

We use the word 'accident' often — 'It was an accident', 'It happened by accident' — almost as though some external force produced the problem and therefore no blame can be attributed to us. In this book we hope to show that many 'accidents' are avoidable either through knowing the possible effects of blows or through knowing what to do. The following accidents relate to real situations:

1. A fifteen-year-old schoolboy loves to watch karate films. One day he playfully chops a school friend on the neck, imitat-

ing a film hero. The friend obligingly drops to the ground just as the film victim did. However, he does not get up again. By the time help arrives the boy's friend is dead.

A statutory post-mortem is carried out and an inquest held. The cause of death is VAGAL CARDIAC INHIBITION and it is confirmed to be due to MISADVENTURE.

2. At a karate competition a competitor sustains a blow to the chest and drops to the floor unconscious. When attempts are made to feel his pulse by the referee it is found to be absent. Several minutes have now elapsed and when experienced help arrives all attempts at cardiac resuscitation are unsuccessful. Death is confirmed to be due to MISADVENTURE and its cause is VAGAL CARDIAC INHIBITION.

3. A young couple are clowning with each other. The young man unintentionally grabs his girlfriend round the neck too strongly and too suddenly. She collapses. He does not know either what to do or what has happened. Unfortunately she is dead when the ambulance arrives. Post-mortem findings imply VAGAL CARDIAC INHIBITION and the death is recorded as due to MISADVENTURE.

These are three tragedies which the term VAGAL CARDIAC INHIBITION as the cause of death in common. This term implies that the heart has suddenly stopped in response to abnormal stimulation of a nerve centre called the VAGUS NERVE (see Fig. 15). There are, of course, other causes of accidental death but we have stressed vagal cardiac inhibition because very little force is required to cause a serious injury and recognition is difficult.

How to avoid disasters

In the disasters already described death occurred because of ignorance of what to do on the part of the observer. Although medical cover is more common now at competitions it is not always available. Combat sports are potentially dangerous activities. Disasters can only be avoided if you are aware that they can happen. Although it is very unlikely that you will ever meet with such a situation you should be prepared to handle it effectively (see Chapter 10). Instructors and members of clubs and associations must be encouraged to take first-aid lessons. With such training yet another facet of your self-confidence will be enhanced.

5.
WOMEN IN COMBAT SPORTS

Women in combat sports are no longer rare birds! Most judo and karate clubs have a large female membership. The sports of kendo, aikido and fencing are also well subscribed.

Before puberty, if the opportunity is given to girls to develop skills in combat, many of them will be stronger and faster than their male counterparts of the same age. Despite the later development of height and weight during puberty, males are often smaller in pre-adolescence and can be as much as two years behind in growth. This advanced physical maturing in girls provides them with an advantage at this stage of development and skills learned can often be superior.

PUBERTY

Girls reach puberty as much as two to three years before their male peers. A girl's mature height is often achieved by a growth spurt at this stage and can be reached shortly after the onset of her periods.

Other changes such as the enlargement of the breasts and increase in body fat may have specific implications for combat training. This increase in body fat means that a female endurance athlete (combat sportswoman) will have a greater proportion of fat to lean body mass (muscle) than a male athlete and the female physique will always remain less angular than that of the lean male.

MENSTRUATION

The onset of periods begins at puberty and continues into late adult life. This single function has led to many misconceptions about training and competition. We must say at this stage that female athletes have won gold medals at every stage of the menstrual cycle, so there is no valid reason why training in females should not be a continuous process throughout each

month as it is in males. Most girls who train accept the occurrence of their periods and although associated with abdominal
discomfort in many, there is evidence to suggest that exercise
during periods is not harmful and may in fact be beneficial.

Sometimes heavy training alone can cause periods to cease.
This is a normal variation in about 15% of female athletes and
does not signify infertility. Another variation is irregularity of
periods caused by training.

Each woman must discover for herself a pattern of training
that is compatible with her menstrual cycle. Usually a regular
training session will suit most.

If periods do not return after giving up training then medical
advice should be sought.

STRENGTH AND ENDURANCE

All available evidence points to the fact that regular exercise will
increase a woman's strength and endurance. Since these are
prerequisites for injury prevention they should be acquired.
There is even some evidence to suggest that women may be
capable of acquiring greater endurance than males.

INJURIES

Most women are less demonstrative about injury than males.
They are no more prone to being injured in combat but there
are specific danger areas.

1. The breasts

The enormous variation in female breast size and shape means
that each individual must take measures 'tailor made' to her
needs in order to avoid injury.

The nipples are especially vulnerable. During body movements the female nipple moves much further than the male.
This makes it prone to inflammation or abrasion. A well-fitting
bra is recommended during training, although some girls are
comfortable wearing no bra.

The breast tissue itself is also likely to be injured from punches or kicks. The most common problem is bruising which

settles well with the ICE regime (see Chapter 9).

The fatty tissue of the breast can however undergo change after a hard punch. The girl notices a firm hard lump some days or weeks after the injury. The medical name for this is FAT NECROSIS. It can occasionally be painful and should always be examined by a doctor. So if a lump appears in your breast, get medical advice. We would suggest that each woman wears a protective brassière of whatever type is comfortable for her.

2. Groin injuries

Although the ovaries, the female reproductive organs, are safely buried deep inside the pelvic cavity, the external genital organs, the vulva and vagina, are liable to injury. Most often lacerations or bruising, which can be quite considerable, will result. Therefore, we suggest that women in combat should wear some form of protection even if it is a sanitary towel. A protective groin guard of the cricket box type is also satisfactory.

3. Special precautions

Dental injury is especially disfiguring for a woman. You should have a gumshield and fight wearing it.

Referees and judges must also ensure that all female competitors have their hair well under control, their nails should be short and they should wear no jewellery. These simple measures will prevent a large number of injuries.

6.
FITNESS, FLEXIBILITY AND STRENGTH IN INJURY PREVENTION

In almost all sports the fittest and most skilful players are least likely to get injured. This is also true in most combat sports. Fitness is an umbrella word used to describe the states of strength, speed, flexibility or staying power of a person. Skill, on the other hand, differentiates a player from others and is both natural or developed by repetition of preset movements. Both skill and fitness are considered in turn.

SKILL IN INJURY PREVENTION

Initially when one learns a combat sport the movements of punching, kicking or throwing are strange and difficult to learn. When sparring after a few months' training, we know what we want to do but somehow cannot put it into practice. Then something happens. With further training and the experience of several fights or competitions under the belt it all becomes so much easier. Before we realise it we have scored a winning throw or punch — or slipped inside a straight left and delivered an overarm right cross in reply. What has happened?

After repeating specific movements time and time again, then coupling this with the experience of fights, movements, initially learned, become automatic. This is the difference between skilled and unskilled fighters. Both think about what they are going to do, but to the skilled man the movements are like reflexes both in attack and defence.

In most scientific studies done on groups of fighters, injuries occur more often when unskilled people fight or spar. Top-class men do also get injuries, but they are not so common, although they are often severe.

So the skill factor is vital in prevention of injury. Every combat sportsperson should aim for a high skill factor. Learn the moves well; practise them often; make them like reflexes.

Physical Fitness

This is a broad term which comprises several components. These are:
1. Flexibility
2. Strength
3. Endurance

All are required in combat sports to some degree.

1. **Flexibility**

This is an aspect of fitness which is sometimes overlooked, but it must never be so. Its role in injury prevention is considered very important. It is an essential part of top-class performance in karate, judo and wrestling. Although different types of flexibility are seen in these sports, they all contribute to preventing injuries, especially to muscles and ligaments. It has been further suggested by training experts in the USA that a degree of overall body flexibility would be a desirable quality for an athlete to possess.

Some of the more appealing aspects of flexibility are:
1. It can be improved by practice.
2. It does not use up energy.
3. It is safe and does not require apparatus.
4. It is enjoyable.

We would recommend that at least fifteen to thirty minutes of flexibility and stretching exercises would be valuable for all combat sports.

Types of flexibility exercise

There are two types: ballistic and static. We prefer the static form because it is much less likely to lead to injury.

Ballistic exercises. You already know these. They involve active exercises usually of the bobbing or bouncing up and down variety. Such exercises *do* stretch the muscles they are meant to, but you do not have such control over them as you do in static stretching. They also lead to a muscle reflex which can actually limit movement.

Static exercises. These are controlled stretching movements.

They can increase the flexibility of the stretched muscle groups if practised only two days a week for thirty minutes. They require little energy and are safe. The exercises are accomplished by SLOWLY moving the body to the stretched position until discomfort is felt. When this happens the stretched

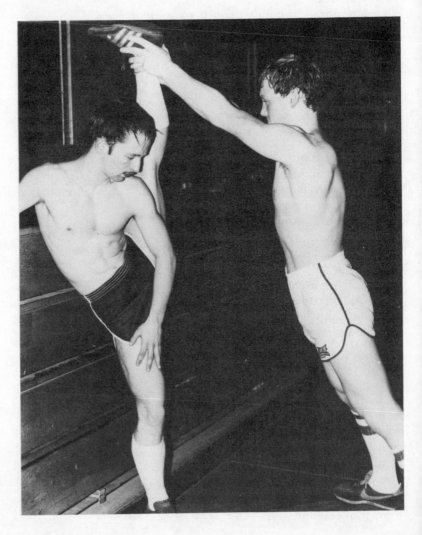

Fig. 12 Flexibility can be acquired and should be done so gradually. Work with a partner whom you can trust.

position is firmly held for up to twenty seconds. Stay relaxed, keep breathing, focus your attention on the part you are stretching.

Train with the assistance of others or alone, but keep variety in your exercises. For instance, you can develop several methods of hamstring or adductor stretching.

2. Strength

Whilst perhaps not so important in punching sports, there is no doubt that strength improves performance in the predominantly grappling sports of judo and wrestling, especially when coupled with skill and experience.

You have all carried out strength exercises in the past and your trainer should be able to design a strength training schedule for you. Basically the requirements for strength development are high resistance and low repetition exercises. Use of slightly heavier weights and lower repetitions than previously used allow muscle bulk and strength to be increased. The training schedule should be at least three days a week — every day if you have the time.

3. Endurance

You are already well aware that staying power in a fight is important. The development of muscular endurance does much to prevent injury. If we examine injury statistics from combat sports it will be seen that injuries are especially liable to occur when an athlete is tiring. This injury situation must be recognised by the referee, for although he cannot stop the fight just because one man is not as fit as the other, he can tighten his control to avoid injury.

In combat, endurance is best built into muscles by circuit training exercises or road-running. If weights are also used in training, the aim should be to use fairly light weights relative to ability and to work fast with high repetitions. Short rests only should be taken between exercises. By doing this, recovery time will eventually be increased.

There is no need to elaborate further on the exercises, for serious athletes are already well aware of what is required. As a coach or trainer of new combat sportsmen your aim should be to instruct them not only in basic skills, but also in endurance exercises. Remember they are not as fit as you. So go easy the first month. If you exhaust your pupils in the first few weeks of training they will not be keen to continue. This will lead to irregular attendances at training and thereby increase the risk of injury. It is sometimes difficult to appreciate how unfit others are, but if you are genuinely interested in your pupils' fitness, welfare and enjoyment of combat sports, you should allow them to make haste . . . slowly!

Recomendations for roadwork

1. Always train wearing comfortable, warm clothing. Unless it is very warm weather, a tracksuit and towel should be worn.
2. If starting roadwork for the first time, or after a long lay-off, run at first on grass and then on roads. Do a short distance every day, or on alternate days, rather than an exhaustive run followed by a long lay-off of several days.
3. Do not run through the pain of injury. This will precipitate chronic problems. Treat muscle or ligament sprains seriously.
4. If you have a cold or minor chest infection, reduce or stop your training until you have recovered. Minor infections can inflame the coverings of the heart and produce abnormal heart rhythms.
5. Consult your trainer if you have any problems. He in turn can discuss them with the club doctor or physiotherapist.
6. Women doing roadwork should wear a well-fitting bra to prevent nipple irritation.

How to assess your fitness

If you are a keen sportsman you will continually wish to improve your cardio-vascular fitness. A number of different training methods are well known to you. These are — circuit training, sprints, distance running, bag work and skipping. They all bring about an increase in heart-lung fitness and increase the body's capacity for supplying oxygen to the muscle cells of the body. This higher capacity for increasing oxygen supply is based on a principle called the LOADING PRIN-

CIPLE. The fighter must apply a work load to his oxygen supply system which is greater than it can cope with easily. In other words it is useless doing long hours of gentle exercise. What is required is short periods of heavy exercise.

The workload you can tolerate depends on how fit you are. You can assess this by pulse counting.

Pulse counting
Feel your pulse on the front of the wrist, just above the skin creases, near the thumb edge of your forearm. Count it for one minute. This is your RESTING PULSE RATE. The increase in pulse rate that you must achieve to improve the function of the oxygen supply system to your muscles — the LOADING PULSE RATE — can be calculated from the following formula:

Necessary increase required equals: 3/5 × (220 minus your age in years minus Resting Pulse Rate).

For example, if you are a 35-year-old sportsman with a Resting Pulse Rate of 60 beats per minute you have to increase your pulse by:

$$\frac{3}{5} \; (220 - 35 - 60)$$

$$= 3 \times \frac{125}{5}$$

$$= 3 \times 25$$

$$= 75 \text{ beats per minute}$$

Therefore you must aim for a pulse rate of 135 to be maintained for at least fifteen minutes per session. This is your LOADING PULSE RATE.

Using this principle the fighter needs only a watch with a second hand to improve his fitness. He can use this principle just as well in a hotel room as in the gym or dojo.

Smoking

One other factor must be mentioned because it can have a significant effect on lung function — cigarette smoking. Much publicity has been given to the serious effects of cigarettes —

lung cancer, heart disease and bronchitis — but regular smoking has other effects which are less serious than these diseases but which impair the lungs' capacity to absorb oxygen. Even in teenagers it is possible to show the effects of cigarettes on lungs' function. This point is worth emphasising particularly for those who work with boys and youths. We do so partly because mild effects in a young smoker can become serious as he grows older, but also because coaches are often looked up to. If a person responsible for boys does not smoke when he is with them, even if he smokes on other occasions, he sets an example which may encourage his lads not to start smoking, resisting the hard man image of the smoker, and may persuade others to stop, or try to stop. It is not easy to stop smoking but it can be done, and the encouragement of his coach may help a boy to do so. Useful advice for someone who wants to stop smoking, or for a person trying to help, is contained in the Health Education Council booklet, *The Smoker's Guide to Non-Smoking*, which should be available free from your health centre or doctor's surgery. (If the receptionist doesn't know of the booklet's existence or whereabouts, ask if you can speak to the health visitor.)

7.
DIET IN SPORT

Diet and athletic performance have always been linked. You only need to scan the sports magazines to see various foodstuffs which guarantee the achievement of your ambitions. The promises are unlimited. It is not surprising then that we often get confused about what to eat and when.

The truth is that a person in good training should eat much the same as everyone else with the addition of extra calories to make up for his energy expenditure. This will involve an adequate intake of carbohydrate, protein and fat. Most vitamins and minerals are available in the foods we eat. However, many athletes take supplements. This does no harm with the exception of Vitamin A. Excess of this vitamin produces acute poisoning.

HOW MANY MEALS?

This is probably a more important question. In training we should eat enough to sustain or even slightly exceed our output. Many authorities now feel that frequent small meals improve athletic performance. This may prove difficult to achieve. We would therefore suggest you eat at least three good meals per day. Breakfast is particularly important.

In training you will require additional calories because of your energy expenditure. This can be achieved by an increase in all aspects of diet but especially in carbohydrate intake.

THREE MAIN FOODS

Food is used as fuel for combustion and the provision of energy as in the motor-car engine. It is also used as building material and for the repair and growth of the tissues. Every living thing has to provide energy to produce activity and maintain body heat. Since body tissues are in constant use, building materials are essential to replace those lost. In children this is especially important since they are actively growing.

Fuel and building materials are not enough. In order that they can be utilised by the tissues we rely on vitamins and water, which is vital for life.

The six essential foods are:

1. Proteins
2. Carbohydrates   } The three main foods
3. Fats
4. Minerals
5. Vitamins
6. Water

All foods contain one or more of these. The body-building foods are proteins, water and salts. The energy producers are carbohydrates and fats. The vitamins and minerals help to make these processes of body building and energy production happen efficiently.

SOURCES OF PARTICULAR FOODS

Protein

Proteins are especially preponderant in the following substances:

Animal proteins	*Vegetable proteins*
Eggs	Wheat and rye
Lean meat	Green vegetables
Milk	Pulses (beans and peas)
Cheese	

Proteins are not generally considered to be an important source of energy although they can be in a state of STAR-VATION. They are needed mainly for building new tissue. You would think that if you wanted to increase muscle size then eating a high-protein diet would be the answer. Not so. We excrete any additional protein eaten if it exceeds 15–20% of dietary intake. So, extra protein is unnecessary.

Fats

This is the energy storehouse in the body. In the average 70 kg person there is 10·5 kg of fat (15% bodyweight). In the highly trained athlete only 5–10% of body weight will be fat.

Dietary fats are available from:

Animal fats	*Vegetable fats*
Fat meat	Oils in margarine
Fish oils	Olive oil
Butter	
Milk and cream	

Fats and carbohydrates provide the source of muscle energy under exercise conditions. How much of each should be in our diet? Generally speaking, during light exercise we rely on fat for muscular energy. As we work harder, carbohydrates become more important. In exhaustive work all muscle energy comes from carbohydrates.

Carbohydrates

These are sugars and starches and make up 45–50% of the total calorie intake. The principal sugar is glucose. Only a limited quantity is stored in the body, in the liver. In exhaustive exercise, if no carbohydrates were taken we would use up the store in two hours. Therefore it is a very important energy source for the combat sportsman. When exhaustion sets in it is usually associated with depleted glucose levels.

Vitamins

These are essential for normal health. Their function is to assist in the utilisation of the main foods. If they are absent from our diet we become ill. The chief vitamins are A, B, C, D, E and K. Vitamins cannot be used as fuel. They are present in small quantities in most foodstuffs.

Vitamin A

Sources Vitamin A is present in animal fats. In carrots and green vegetables a substance is found which the body converts to Vitamin A.

Deficiency causes lowered resistance to infection, stunted growth, eye complaints.

Vitamin B complex

Sources Yeast, yeast extracts, cereals, vegetables, fruit, milk, eggs, meats.

Deficiency causes nervous disorders, constipation, tingling and burning of the feet, skin disorders, blood disorders.

Vitamin C

Sources Citrus fruits (oranges, grapefruit, lemons), blackcurrants, green peppers, potatoes.

Deficiency causes scurvy (a bleeding condition in which skin blood vessels become fragile and burst).

Vitamin D

Sources Cod liver oil, halibut oil, animal fats. Sunlight allows vitamin D to be made in the skin.

Deficiency causes bone disorders — rickets in children, soft bones in adults.

Vitamin E

Sources Vegetable oils.

Deficiency No known symptoms.

Vitamin K

Sources Green vegetables, liver.

Deficiency causes bleeding tendencies.
NB Vitamin K is also synthesised in the intestines by bacteria.

We can see that deficiency of vitamins is unlikely to occur with the usual mixed diet eaten in this country. Most experts are in agreement that there is no need to take additional vitamins in the form of supplements. However, provided the amount taken is not excessive this will cause no harm.

Minerals

These are present in many foods. Their absence can produce a range of symptoms from nausea and vomiting to extreme muscular weakness. They have diverse functions: they regulate tissue activity and carry electrical charges which allow normal metabolism to continue.

Sodium is obtained from animal foodstuffs and cooking salt. Its depletion is especially likely when heavy sweating occurs over a prolonged period. Another cause of loss is a humid warm atmosphere. Sodium loss produces excessive fatigue and muscular cramps. Tennis players are at risk and you will have seen them take salt tablets between games.

Unless you sweat profusely over a very long period depletion is unlikely.

Potassium is obtained from plant foodstuffs. Its depletion can result in profound muscle weakness. In combat sport this would be a very unlikely occurrence in an otherwise healthy person.

Calcium is the commonest mineral in the body. It is an important constituent of bones and teeth. Apart from this it plays important roles in the clotting of blood and in controlling the action of the heart and skeletal muscles.

It is found in milk, cheese and hard water. Defiency leads to rickets in children and softening of the bones in adults. The latter is unlikely in the fit athlete.

Iron Most iron is derived from eggs, meat, green vegetables and fish. Liver has a high iron content.

Iron is necessary for the blood pigment — HAEMO-GLOBIN. This is the important oxygen carrier in the blood.

Deficiency of iron leads to anaemia, which can produce fatigue and poor training performance.

Phosphorus is present in large amounts in the bones and teeth. It also has a part to play in the absorption of carbohydrates.

Deficiency is very unlikely. Phosphorus is present in meats, fish, eggs and cereals.

Iodine is present in sea foods and vegetables. It plays an important part in normal metabolism through the thyroid gland in the neck. Its deficiency produces slowing of body metabolism and mental processes. This was particularly likely to happen in certain areas of Britain — especially Derbyshire — where iodine sources were lacking because of certain factors in the soil or water. Iodised salt is available on demand.

There are in addition many other minerals which are vital for normal function. However, it would be rare to discover a mineral deficiency in combat sportsmen.

Water

About 70% of our body weight is water. It is vital and involved in almost every bodily function in some way. A constant supply is essential. It is lost in the faeces, sweat and breath. Thirst ensures an adequate supply. If water is withheld for a few days in a fast, death will result. People on long fasts can survive many weeks provided water is available.

Depletion is temporary in training and replenished with drinks.

THE TRAINING DIET

Combat sportsmen are endurance athletes. You will have to cope with a high rate of energy expenditure both in training and contest. A well-balanced mixed diet is essential. It should contain 15–20% protein; 30–40% fats and 45–50% carbohydrates. Such a diet will also contain enough vitamins and minerals.

Carbohydrate loading

Chronic muscular exhaustion can result from an extremely strenuous regime of training. Scientific studies have shown that this is related to depletion of a carbohydrate complex which is present in the muscles. This is called GLYCOGEN. When muscles are very active it supplies energy. After two to three days of long distance runs (more than 10 miles a day) the glycogen in muscle is reduced to near zero. It has been shown that even a high carbohydrate diet will not replace this quickly despite rest. What distance runners do to achieve excellent performance for a big race is to eat only proteins and fats in their diet for several days of heavy training. This depletes muscle glycogen. They then ingest a very high carbohydrate diet for three to four days to coincide with the race. This is a common practice in runners. If you have problems with stamina in a long fight (ten to fifteen rounds) this may be worth trying. Do it only with the help of an experienced dietitian.

IT IS MOST UNLIKELY THAT THE AVERAGELY-TRAINED FIGHTER WILL REQUIRE SUCH A REGIME. THERE IS NO EVIDENCE TO SHOW THAT CARBO-HYDRATE LOADING IMPROVES PERFORMANCE IN EVENTS OF UNDER THIRTY MINUTES.

Making the weight

Weight reduction

This should be achieved by a reduction in body fat and ideally should be at a rate of 1 kg (2.2 lb) per week. The fighter should therefore aim for his 'ideal' weight two to three weeks (or more) before his fight. The safe way to achieve this is through a modest dietary reduction and a modest increase in training. Starvation and rapid dehydration compromise performance through weakness and impaired endurance. Ask your general practitioner for a diet sheet. Do not take fluid-depleting drugs. They can have serious consequences.

Gaining weight

The aim should be to increase muscle mass. Weight gain may be important for judoka and wrestlers. Fat increases only can lead to complications.

Muscle mass can be increased by heavy muscle training in the form of weight-training and increased food intake. This increase in food should be low in fat but high in carbohydrate. It can be effectively achieved by eating two extra snacks a day.

Anabolic steroids

Although widely used these drugs are regarded as unethical in sport. It is inevitable that you may be tempted to take them if you wish rapid weight gain. As the rules stand you run a risk of being disqualified for cheating. Remember too that the long-term risks may outweigh any short-term benefits. We would strongly advise you *not* to take steroids. However, if you must, it is wise to consult a doctor regularly. He will be unlikely to prescribe steroids for you, but surveillance is essential. Our advice may cause adverse comments. However, we feel steroids are taken widely and if you do take them you may be at risk from effects of overdosage. Consult the doctor. The relationship between you and him is confidential.

Fluid intake

We have mentioned loss of salt during sweating. Most sweat is water but potassium can also be lost. In a strenuous session in a warm environment as much as two litres of water may be lost.

Replacement should be regular throughout the training session. Small amounts of cool fluid are best. In an actual fight only a mouthful should be swallowed in each round. Start the fight well hydrated and a mouth wash only will be required.

We would recommend that you use only water in a fight. A very small quantity of glucose should be added with flavouring such as orange juice during training sessions. Small quantities are advised.

After the session, modest salt addition to your food will replace any losses.

What to eat before the contest

A steak before the contest is not advisable. It slows the emptying of the stomach and may take three or four hours to be digested. Fatty food should also be avoided.

If you must eat a proper meal make sure it is high in calories from carbohydrates and that it is taken at least three hours before the contest.

The ideal pre-contest 'meal' would be liquid containing no gas and high in carbohydrates. A weak glucose-containing drink would provide this.

One further tip. A cup of coffee is thought to contain just enough caffeine to increase energy production in the body by allowing fats to be used efficiently. This is not doping and you may find it effective.

8.
BEFORE THE BELL — AFTER THE BELL

In this short chapter we discuss the 'taboo' areas for sportsmen and, we hope, explode some of the myths.

ALCOHOL

Most people in Britain drink alcohol and there is no evidence to show that moderate alcoholic intake hampers progress unduly. Drinking to excess, however, will cause marked deterioration in performance. Athletes are people who suffer stress just like everyone else. The coach should therefore take note if an athlete's performance is deteriorating and inquire into his/her problems. It may be that the sportsman will be more prepared to discuss his worries with the coach than with a doctor. Often alcohol is used to relieve stress and it may be the symptom of an underlying depression.

When training for an important fight alcohol is usually forbidden. This is very sensible and if the athlete can tolerate this imposed discipline it will probably improve his all-round fitness and prepare him better psychologically. An occasional pint of beer, however, if he can't cope, will not ruin his chances of success completely.

SEX

There are many myths both for and against sexual intercourse in relation to physical performance. Some top athletes have boasted that they compete better after intercourse. There are no rules regarding this. Certainly all available evidence suggests that neither abstinence nor indulgence will hamper performance in sport.

One famous American baseball player was notorious for his interest in girls before a match. He used to say, 'It's not going to bed with a woman that makes a ballplayer play badly, it's staying up all night looking for one that makes him shattered!'

So the motto is 'Do what you like' but get yourself properly organised!

SLEEP

All training athletes need sleep. It assists digestion and allows injuries to heal. Its relaxant effect also lets tired muscles recover.

Before a major contest you should not break your sleeping pattern by going to bed early. Get into a routine during training. Ensure that you get at least eight hours' sleep per night. This is the average requirement. Some people will require a little more or less.

Remember, too, that sleepiness can be a sign that you are overtraining. If you find yourself napping at work or at odd times throughout the day you may be overdoing it. Review your training schedule and make any necessary alterations after discussion with your coach.

DRUGS

Strength athletes are especially prone to abuse drugs. Wrestlers or judoka may also be encouraged to do so in order to compete at higher weights.

The most commonly abused are the anabolic steroids. They are said to increase weight, strength and speed by increasing aggression, allowing more training sessions and causing retention of body water. Most athletes who take them overdose themselves grossly. The side effects vary from acne and dizziness at one end of the spectrum to diabetes and liver cancer at the other. Women may experience deeping of the voice and facial hair growth. Child athletes who take such drugs run a high risk of their growth being stunted, for the steroid drugs can lead to premature fusion of the growing ends of the bones.

The rules are quite clear regarding the use of such agents and all other drugs not prescribed by a doctor (even some prescribed by a doctor). Any athlete who takes such drugs to assist performance is guilty of cheating and will not be allowed to compete in his event. He even runs the risk of being banned completely.

MINOR ILLNESS

Colds or coughs with runny nose symptoms occur from time to time. We advise you to reduce your training intensity during such minor illnesses or even to lay off altogether. Our reason is simple. Minor viral illnesses can produce inflammation of the membrane covering the heart. This can lead to abnormal rhythms, especially during exercise. Sudden death in young athletes has *occasionally* been due to this condition. The viruses producing minor respiratory symptoms are often attracted also to the heart membrane.

RETIRING FROM COMBAT SPORT

Only a few exceptional athletes continue to compete into middle age. This is one of the sad facts about sport. What do you do when you stop competing?

The problem arises only in boxing, judo and wrestling to any real degree. The martial arts have a slightly different philosophy in that progress continues even into old age. Funakoshi Gichin is reported to have said to one of his disciples at the age of eighty plus that he was only now beginning to feel the true 'Tsuki'. This is a sound concept which can be effectively applied to all sport.

When you retire from the competition for good, a gap is left which you may be unable to fill. You should consider this even while you are still competing. Various avenues are open to you such as continuing to train, refereeing, coaching, judging, improving standards for other fighters, working for sponsorship, etc. We believe you should plan your future and maintain your interests. This is another form of prevention. Retired sportsmen can suddenly become very fat, depressed people. Try to stay active and interested in others! You may surprise yourself by discovering how rewarding this can be.

9.
ABOUT INJURIES

UNDERSTANDING INJURIES

A rational approach to injury management requires a basic understanding of the injury process. Irrespective of where an injury occurs in the body the same processes of repair and healing take place. Depending on what tissue is injured the rates will differ. With few exceptions — muscular and nervous tissue — the original tissue is reformed after an injury.

When tissue damage occurs it is usually accompanied by some bleeding. This is added to by tissue fluid. These contribute to the *swelling* so often seen after injury and also account in part for *pain* since the damaged and swollen tissue stimulates nerve endings in the area. In addition the swelling makes the injured part stiff preventing further use. This LOSS OF FUNCTION allows reparative processes to begin to work and prevents re-injury. Finally, the increased bleeding and tissue fluid make the area both *warm* and usually *reddened*. These are the five characteristics of inflammation and physical injury produces exactly that. What should be done to limit such inflammation?

Initial treatment for these and most injuries to skin, muscles and bones is described throughout this book as the ICE regime.

Ice should be applied to cause contraction of the blood vessels round the injured part which reduces swelling and bleeding.

Compression also prevents excessive swelling.

Elevation reduces the flow of blood to the injured part.

INJURY PREVENTION

Prevention through protective clothing

Protective clothing in the form of headgear and kidney and groin guards is encourged in boxing sparring. Many forms of padding are now available in karate and are discussed in another

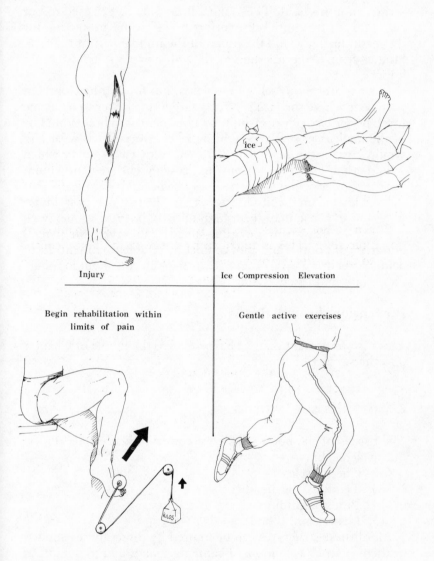

Injury

Ice Compression Elevation

Begin rehabilitation within limits of pain

Gentle active exercises

Fig. 13 The ICE regime and rehabilitation.

part of this book. Remember that the purpose of training and sparring is to sharpen your techniques for the fight proper. If you can avoid injury you will perform confidently in the contest.

In the punching and kicking combat sports it is advisable to wear a mouth guard. They take a little time to get used to but make up for this initial discomfort by affording protection for the teeth, lips, jaw and the bones of the middle part of the face. Studies from America suggest they also protect against being knocked out.

Most sports shops sell gum-shields, but for combat sports in particular where the face is often a target it is better to have one (even better two) custom-built by your dentist. These would be of the malleable, soft type which are comfortable to wear and would cost in the region of £15 — £25 for two shields which would last at least two seasons. In growing children and young people regular dental inspection may be necessary to ensure that the shield remains well-tailored. Your dentist will best advise you. The expense may seem high initially but it is money well spent. The £25 spent on gum-shields can save you several hundreds of pounds and a lot of uncomfortable treatment. Each dentist's fee for a gum-shield will vary but you should arrange to see him and discuss your needs.

Prevention through fitness

This is so important that we have devoted the whole of Chapter 6 to the subject of fitness.

COMMON TISSUE INJURIES

The tissues of the body which are commonly affected are:
1. The skin
2. The muscles
3. Tendons and ligaments
4. Bones and joints
5. Nerves and blood vessels

All of these structures can be injured by direct forces applied to them. Muscles, tendons, ligaments, bones and joints can in addition suffer from injuries which we group together under the term 'overuse injuries'. These injuries are in many cases exclusive to athletes who in trying to achieve superlative performance push their bodies to the limit and often beyond.

All injuries should be treated as early as possible in order to get good results and the treatment regimes are described in detail throughout the book. We must stress, however, that overuse injuries are sometimes extremely resistant to treatment. You should not feel that it is giving in to refer an athlete early to his doctor for what may be an apparently minor twinge such as pain in his Achilles tendon every time he runs. Overuse injuries can be debilitating and will produce long lay-offs from training if they become chronic. THEREFORE IF THE INJURIES (detailed subsequently) DO NOT RESPOND TO TREATMENT WITHIN FORTY-EIGHT HOURS, GET MEDICAL ADVICE THAT WEEK.

OVERUSE PROBLEMS IN CHILDREN AND ADOLESCENTS

Children and adolescents must be treated by the instructor as a special group. Their bones have not yet finished growing and their muscles and tendons are not yet firmly bound to their bony attachments in many sites of the body. Until growth stops, all young people under 18 years old can suffer from a specific group of injuries called 'adolescent overuse injuries'. These can produce chronic pain in training but more importantly permanent damage to bone or muscle. As a responsible teacher their safety is your concern.

The injuries affect special sites — usually the elbow, the hips and groin, the tibial tubercle (the bump at the upper end of the shin bone into which the patellar tendon is attached), the knee-cap itself, the knee joint and the bones of the foot and hand.

The symptoms are of persistent pain at these sites, sometimes with deformity, swelling and tenderness. DO NOT ATTEMPT TO TREAT INJURIES SUCH AS THESE YOURSELF. Make certain the child or young person's parents are informed and advise the need for a medical opinion.

SKIN

Skin and subcutaneous tissue form a waterproof insulation for the body. Skin is tough, elastic and can be deformed easily. It is especially prone to injury when compressed against a bony surface (such as around the eye socket or bridge of the nose or over the cheek bones). Shearing forces can also produce injury. Most heal well, but regard all with respect. If the cut opens again it could cause you to lose your next fight.

Bruises occur as a result of direct trauma — a punch, kick or continued sustained pressure. They can be quite extensive. They are due to bleeding from small blood vessels. As time passes the bruise may actually enlarge because the blood spreads under the skin. So a black eye may be even more unsightly after three days than at first.

Abrasions and lacerations An abrasion or graze occurs after a glancing blow (the punch you slipped, almost!) Although painful, they heal quickly. Lacerations involve damage to the whole skin thickness. They can be simple cuts when the edges are well defined or they can be star-shaped with ragged edges.

Blisters are also common and troublesome. They occur in the hands and feet (sometimes the knee in wrestlers and judoka). They are produced by recurrent minor shearing stresses which strip one layer of skin from the one underneath. They are painful. If the area is repeatedly subjected to frictional stress the end result is a protective CALLOSITY.

Prevention of skin problems

Whenever the skin is broken the possibility of infection arises. One particularly severe infection is TETANUS or LOCKJAW. This is produced by bacteria usually present in the soil but by no means unknown or indoor floors. Therefore immunisation against tetanus is worthwhile since it is difficult to treat. Immunisation can also be given by your own doctor or in hospital within twenty-four hours of injury. A course consists of three injections, the second to be carried out six weeks after the first, and the third approximately six months later. A booster injection is then required every five years thereafter.

Treatment of injuries to the skin

Bruises should be treated by applying crushed ice in a pack or a chemical ice pack.

Abrasions. These scraping injuries to the skin may vary in severity from a simple graze to very extensive damage. Areas commonly injured include the shin, the knee, the pelvic crest (felt below the ribs on each side), the elbow and the back of the hand. Abrasions are not in themselves serious but if extensive you must ascertain that there is no damage to underlying structures such as nerve, tendon or bone. If there is any doubt a MEDICAL OPINION should be sought immediately. We cannot overemphasise the need to care for any break in the skin because of the risk of TETANUS INFECTION.

In simple abrasions the skin should be cleaned with *soap and water* or a mild antiseptic such as *Dettol*. Ground-in dirt can be brushed out with a soft brush (soft clean nailbrush). This will prevent subsequent tatooing which is staining of the skin due to imbedded foreign material.

Once the wound is clean it should be gently dried with a clean towel and a dry dressing applied daily when training. This acts as a protection against further injury. Otherwise the area should be exposed to the air. Most abrasions heal quickly and well. If infection supervenes contact your doctor.

Burns should be treated along the same lines as abrasions. If the burns are extensive, medical care is mandatory. If they are limited, leave the burned area exposed to the air as much as possible and apply a dry protective dressing only when training. It may also give some relief to keep a burn covered in the early stages after it has occurred. Otherwise it should be left open to the air.

Lacerations require accurate approximation of the skin edges. This is best achieved by sutures (stitches) or steristrip (skin plasters). In this way a broad scar is prevented. These are liable to break down again if further traumatised as invariably will happen in boxing. You may have had this experience. Many well-known boxers have had a 'cut' problem. Some have even required plastic surgical techniques to get a good repair.

Blisters can be treated in two ways. One is to rest and stop doing the action which causes them. This takes time. The most effective method is to puncture the blister with a sterile needle but to leave the blistered skin which acts as a biological dressing. Clean the area with antiseptic and apply zinc oxide plaster. Aseptic principles must be observed to prevent infection.

Complications of infections of cuts and abrasions

Prevention of tetanus infection should be paramount. This is effectively acquired by immunisation.

Other infections can occur in wounds or abrasions. One of these is CELLULITIS. This is caused by bacteria which can digest skin proteins and therefore the infection spreads through the skin. Recognise it by the following signs:

1. The fighter will have sustained a cut or graze.
2. The area around will become reddened and swollen within twenty-four to forty-eight hours.
3. There will be considerable throbbing; even pain and healing will be delayed.
4. The area itself will be tender to touch, and the skin will appear reddened around the area injured. This may extend along a limb for a considerable distance.
5. The person may begin to feel physically ill.

If these signs develop it is essential to see your doctor. He may prescribe ANTIBIOTICS. Take them exactly as he states and complete the course even if you feel better. If you get a rash or feel nauseated return to your doctor, as these are fairly common side effects (unpleasant symptoms associated with antibiotics).

PERSONAL HYGIENE

If you do not keep your gear clean you will run the risk of infection from a fungus and may suffer from athlete's foot or groin (jock-itch). These problems are common to all combat sports and are highly infectious.

The conditions present as an irritating itch between the toes or in the groin crease. Spread is through direct contact with floors, shower rooms and other moist surfaces which actually harbour the infection and spread it from person to person. Using the same towel all week, sharing towels or wearing a dirty groin guard contribute to the infection.

Prevention of fungus infections

You should, if possible, have two (or even three) sets of training gear so that one set is always regularly laundered. This is one very important aspect of prevention.

If only one set of training gear is available it should be washed as regularly as possible — at least twice a week — and allowed to dry overnight. In this way you can ensure that your gear is always fresh.

Coaches and trainers involved with children or adolescents should give advice to parents either personally or through a club card of 'do's and don'ts for karate, aikido, boxing, etc.' to make certain that fresh gear will be in use. It may even be possible for arrangements to be made through the clubs to have gear laundered, in the same way as football kit is. This would ensure they were fresh at least once a week.

We cannot overstress the importance of fresh kit. Parents and coaches must take this responsibility seriously. Young men and women in combat sport must also make certain that this important aspect of personal hygiene is not ignored.

Adequate foot care is also essential for the prevention of athlete's foot. This means washing your feet at least once a day and certainly after every training session. Wash them quickly in warm water. Do not soak them for long periods. Dry them gently and leave them exposed for several minutes before putting on your socks, which should be changed daily. In all combat sports foot care is vital but very often ignored. The use of talcum powder once the feet are dry is refreshing but is no substitute for proper drying, especially between the toes. Your daily socks are also important. Nylon socks actually increase sweating. We would recommend woollen or synthetic non-nylon socks.

Treatment of athlete's foot and groin is with anti-fungal preparations such as MYCIL or TINADERM. These are available from your chemist without prescription. If there is no improvement in two weeks consult your doctor. Prevent the spread of athlete's foot to others by standing on a towel after showering. This towel should be used for no other purpose. Do not walk with bare feet on surfaces used by other fighters. Obviously this may mean that you should not train barefoot. You should discuss this with your teacher.

Athlete's groin should be treated in a similar fashion. Use a separate towel to dry the groin creases and keep your groin support clean.

Verrucas and corns

Barefoot fighters, like swimmers, can get virus infections of their feet which cause foot warts (verrucas). This always occurs on the sole of the foot and it feels as though one is walking on a pebble. It requires specialist treatment, either from a doctor or a chiropodist. Any barefoot fighter with a verruca should explain to his coach that he has the condition and should be allowed to train wearing light plimsolls. He should also bathe separately and wear plastic sandals in the shower.

A corn is thickening of normal skin in relation to friction from shoes, usually due to pressure points. It can be successfully treated with lanolin and abrading it with an emery board (a cardboard nail file).

One further point in prevention of infection is to keep your finger and toe nails short and clean. Long nails can produce cuts which may result in painful infection.

It is also vital that hair is kept short at the front or well tied back, since good vision — especially a wide field of vision — is essential for a fighter. Boxers' hair must be kept short.

MUSCLES

Injury to muscle can produce symptoms ranging from a minor 'twinge' on movement which settles with time to severe pain and fear brought on every time an exercise or movement is performed.

Each muscle is described as having an ORIGIN and an INSERTION (Fig. 14). The origin can be from bone, or tendon-like structures. The insertion is into bone or tendon beyond the next joint. In between is the muscle BELLY which is made up of muscle fibres arranged in parallel. Each fibre can contract, and when mass contraction of fibres occurs the muscle produces movement of the joint. Most of the time we use only 40–50 per cent of all the muscle fibres in each muscle. Combat training allows us to use more than this at will. This is why the effects of combat skills can be so devastating.

The importance of warm-up

Warm-up is poorly understood, even by doctors, but there is

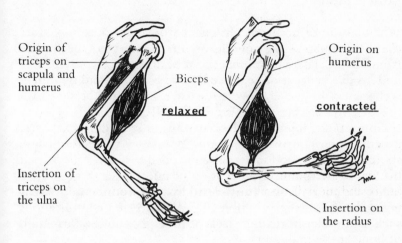

Origin of triceps on scapula and humerus

Biceps

relaxed

Origin on humerus

contracted

Insertion of triceps on the ulna

Insertion on the radius

Fig. 14 The origin and insertion of a muscle. When the biceps contracts it flexes the elbow and rotates the forearm outwards. The brachialis muscle lies near the origin of the biceps.

little doubt that it reduces the risk of injury and improves performance. It increases the speed and force of muscular contraction, and when related to the particular activity about to be undertaken it seems to sharpen co-ordination. Especially important in endurance combat sports is the fact that proper warm-up brings on second wind more readily.

The requirements for adequate warm-up are that:

1. It should be intense enough to produce perspiration but not so intense that it causes partial fatigue.
2. It should include loosening and stretching exercises.
3. It should include movements such as shadow boxing, blocks, etc. so as to improve co-ordination for the fight itself.
4. It should taper off so that it ends about five minutes before the fight. This will allow recovery from any slight fatigue.

REMEMBER: Keep warm after warm-up. Wear a track suit, jersey or dressing-gown and towel.

Muscle injury

When an injury occurs it can result from two causes — either over-stretching of the muscle or direct injury to the muscle from blows. The whole muscle can be affected, or only part of it. This difference is of degree only and basic first-aid treatment is the same. However, severe muscle tears should be seen by a doctor — ON THE DAY OF THE INJURY.

Commonly, injuries will occur during stretching exercises, usually when poorly warmed-up. You should therefore begin stretching slowly and in a well-controlled manner, especially if the training hall is cold.

Muscle injury is usually attended by pain, considerable swelling and stiffness. Early action PREVENTS later complications such as muscle shortening, lack of mobility and the formation of bone at the injury site.

How to treat muscle injuries

Immediate application of an ice pack for five to seven minutes until the skin turns pink will relieve pain and swelling. If a limb is involved, elevate it. Apply a tubigrip bandage and reapply the ice pack every ten minutes through the bandage. The first few hours are vital if recovery is to be complete. The injured person should also take an analgesic (pain killer) such as ASPIRIN in these early stages.

Obviously a major tear is best treated at a hospital where follow-up may include physiotherapy. Forty-eight hours after a muscle injury is the average time taken to start remobilisation. After this time most pain has settled and active exercise within the limits of pain can be started.

Complications of muscle injury

Infection is uncommon in muscle injuries. Sometimes intra-muscular cysts form if the muscle bleeding does not settle adequately. A cyst is a sac inside the muscle. It contains fluid and is best treated by a doctor.

Shortening of the muscle is always a problem after injury.

This occurs because muscle tissue heals by forming fibrous tissue which is inelastic. The rehabilitation of a muscle injury must therefore include stretching exercises to regain length and flexibility.

Bone formation

It is a bad move to massage a thigh injury. In many cases the blood clot will increase in size and may become hardened with calcium or even form a mass of bone. This condition has been known for many years. It is disabling and difficult to treat. It can occur in any thigh injury but is especially common when the thigh is massaged after injury. Thigh injuries must be treated with respect, otherwise a prolonged period off sport will result and perhaps even surgical treatment may be required.

Local gangrene

In those styles of karate (such as Kyokushinkai) where frequent sweeps or low leg kicks are used, the risk of this condition increases. The group of muscles just to the side of the shin are involved. When bruised from kicks they swell, but unlike other muscles they are enclosed in a tight compartment by fibrous tissue. The swelling compresses the artery which supplies blood to the area and can occlude it. So gangrene can result. Any fighter who complains of tingling in the spaces between the toes with pain just to the side of the shin should be stopped, the leg elevated and ice packs applied. Hospital opinion is necessary if pain remains unrelieved after more than twenty minutes of this treatment.

Tendons And Ligaments

Tendons are fibrous bands which connect muscles to bones. Ligaments are fibrous bands which support joints. Tendons may become inflamed due to overuse. An example is the Achilles tendon in runners. Tendons can also be partially or completely torn.

Ligaments can be stretched leading to partial or complete tearing. The word *sprain* is usually applied to minor tears of the ligament. These injuries result from twisting or wrenching of the affected joints.

Tendonitis

When a tendon or its coverings become inflamed this is called TENDONITIS. In combat sports the triceps tendon (from punching without a target), the tendons in the shoulder (same reason), the Achilles tendon (from roadwork) and the adductor tendons on the inside of the thigh (from over-vigorous stretching) are the commonest tendons involved.

Treatment involves rest — and this is one area where rest is vital — ultrasonic therapy and anti-inflammatory drugs (prescribed by the club doctor). Usually the problem settles. Again, carefully planned treatment when symptoms appear is the key. If tendon pain occurs, all activity should be stopped and the ICE regime begun. Rehabilitation should be gradual with graded exercise over several weeks.

Ligaments

Partial or complete tears all require medical treatment, often surgery. The diagnosis is not difficult. There is extreme pain, swelling over the affected joint and instability of the joint. Severe symptoms should arouse your suspicions. Physiotherapy and retraining are required post-operatively.

Sprains are diagnosed by the presence of tenderness over the ligaments on either side of a joint. Finger-joint ligament sprains are common in fighters. Treat these injuries with ice and strapping to the other finger. This will allow the fighter to carry on. He should continue ice treatment after the fight is over. Contrast bathing (hot and cold water) will also help the swelling to settle.

BONES AND JOINTS

In all collision sports there is a chance of a bone or joint injury. Most often it is those bones which lie just under the skin which cause problems. Feel down your shin bones. It is called the tibia. Put your hand flat on the table and feel the bone of your forearm from your elbow down to your hand. This is the ulna. The tibia can be bruised or broken when legs clash or kicks are blocked by the arm (when the ulna is also injured!)

Other bones can be damaged too. In punches the thumb bones and wrist bones can be put at risk from accidental collisions or poorly delivered blows. The ribs are also especially vulnerable to damage. A broken rib makes it painful to breathe and cough.

One other type of bone injury can occur. It is called a 'stress' fracture. It affects the tibia most often and can be a cause of pain in that bone. It is especially prevalent amongst fighters who do a lot of roadwork to stay fit and is one of the many causes of the condition called 'shin splints' (Chapter 18).

How to deal with injuries to bone

This chapter is designed only to acquaint you with the kind of injury which can occur. Full details are given later. Briefly, when there is bone pain, suspect a fracture (break), especially if the person cannot weight-bear on the affected leg and there is local tenderness. If the arm is affected, tenderness over the injury site and painful movements suggest fracture. Hospital advice and X-ray are required — AT THE TIME OF INJURY, not two or three days later. If transport is uncomfortable, bandage the injured leg to its neighbour or put the arm in a sling until hospital is reached (Chapters 17, 18).

Joints

Joints are of three types:
1. BONE TO BONE, e.g. the flat bones that make up the skull.
2. BONE — FIBROUS TISSUE — BONE, e.g. the junction of the bones of the pelvis.
3. BONE — FLUID MEMBRANE — BONE, e.g. the knee, the shoulder, the elbow, etc.

You will have realised already that the types of joint in 1 and 2 do not move — unless they sustain injury. The joint most often injured is type 3. Because these joints move freely they must gain strength from ligaments and muscles. These, too, can be torn in injury.

Types of joint injury

A force deforming a joint can dislocate it. That means the joint is actually pulled out of its socket and will not return unless the dislocation is reduced. Less severe injuries can produce breaks in the bones around the joint or cracks and loose bone fragments inside the joint cavity. All of these injuries demand hospital management — AT THE TIME OF INJURY.

How to manage a joint injury

There will be severe pain which may frighten you, for your injured colleague will grimace in agony. Gently support the affected joint and help to place it in the most comfortable position. Once this is achieved, bandage the arm to the body or the one leg to the other. DON'T DELAY HOSPITAL TRANSFER, as some joint injuries can damage important blood vessels in a limb.

NERVES AND BLOOD VESSELS

Nerves are like electric cables which relay messages from the brain or spinal cord to muscle and skin. They are prone to injury in the neck, the arms and legs. The vagus nerve is most important — this is discussed in Chapter 10. Two nerves in the arm and one in the leg are commonly injured in combat. Another nerve which gives sensation to the skin below the eye produces numbness below the eye when the cheek bone is broken. The signs and symptoms produced are detailed in the chapters on the specific parts of the body.

How to deal with nerve injuries

The vagus nerve needs special treatment. Injure it and you may have to perform cardiac massage. Fortunately the others are not so dramatic. The symptoms settle with rest but if you suspect a broken arm or leg don't hesitate to get medical help.

Nerve pain can last from minutes to weeks. Be reassured, though, it almost always settles.

REHABILITATION AFTER INJURY

Rehabilitation aims to restore normal function after injury. When applied to non-athletes it may be said to be complete when the injured person can re-use the injured part. Athletes, however, not only wish return of function but also hope to have *return of previous performance*. The injured area should be progressively encouraged to take a little more strain as each day passes. Reference to the previous day's performance is also essential to ensure progress.

Rehabilitation should start straight away. Ease the pain and limit swelling using the ICE regime. Usually within twelve to twenty-four hours gentle movements can be begun (excluding broken bones, of course!) but always within the limits of pain. If, for example, an adductor sprain has recurred, stretching exercises should be performed very gradually to maintain flexibility. Never suddenly overload the injury. Medical or physiotherapy advice should be understood and religiously followed.

Another aspect of rehabilitation is maintaining fitness whilst injured. To achieve this, design a series of exercises which exclude the injured part. They should be strenuous enough to cause breathlessness. By maintaining general fitness, confidence is also kept high. Such exercises could include sit-ups, chinning the bar, press-ups, air cycling (lying on the back), performing cycling movements of the leg and swimming (an excellent method), depending on the area injured.

Only when full movements with the affected areas are pain-free is return to normal training possible.

THE NEED FOR MEDICAL ADVICE

Finally, in all combat sports we feel it is necessary to have access to a doctor familiar with sports injuries. He represents the ultimate defence against mismanagement of injuries and even tragedy on occasions. Furthermore several members of the club — preferably coaches and referees — should try to acquire first-aid training. It would not be regretted.

10.
EMERGENCY SITUATIONS

How To Stay Cool

In almost every combat sport an emergency will arise at some time. This might involve unconsciouness, the suspicion of a neck injury, a broken bone, bleeding or even cardiac arrest. The best way to stay cool is to anticipate such a situation and take the responsibility on yourself of acquiring first-aid skills. Even with these skills you might feel anxious but certainly not so afraid as when you are totally ignorant and quite unable to help. At your club, therefore, members should be encouraged to get first-aid training by attending sessions run by the local first-aid group or doctor.

With such knowledge you will be able to handle most emergency situations which arise in combat sport effectively. Further, it is essential that you control the spectators when such an incident arises. Often the crowding onlookers can hamper attempts at treatment by giving all kinds of advice. If you know what to do you will not have to listen to them. Make certain that you have adequate space by requesting that spectators keep well clear by returning to their seats in an orderly fashion.

First-Aid Equipment

First-aid and adequate equipment are the basics of injury control. The club should have a first-aid bag, the contents of which should include:
1. Crepe bandages — 4″ and 6″ — two of each
2. Elastoplast bandages — 4″ and 6″ — two of each
3. Slings — triangular bandages for upper limb injuries — two of each
4. Eye pad, vision card, pen torch
5. Elastoplast dressings, heavy-duty scissors, micropore tape
6. Antiseptic solutions, e.g. Dettol, povidone-iodine solution (Napp Laboratories)

7. Ice packs, either chemical or in plastic bags from the fridge
8. Cotton wool, gauze swabs, assorted surgical tapes
9. Aspirin or paracetamol. Other anti-inflammatory agents can be prescribed by your doctor.

In addition, the following may be required for competitions and should be used only by TRAINED PERSONS:

1. Oral airways — small, medium and large
2. Stretcher (rigid foldable), sandbags
3. Inflatable, rigid splints

Remember, after administering first aid, to get the severely injured player or fighter to a hospital for definitive care.

How To Recognise A Fracture

A fracture is a break, usually in a bone. It can be SIMPLE or COMPOUND. In a simple fracture the skin is unbroken by the bone ends. The break may be a hairline crack or there may be marked displacement of the broken bones with resultant limb deformity.

A compound fracture, on the other hand, implies that the skin has been broken by the bone ends which may protrude through it. Sometimes a puncture wound is all that is seen. When a fracture is compound, infection can get into the bone. This must always be regarded as a serious injury, as bony infections can be very difficult to eradicate.

Signs and symptoms

A fracture is usually followed by pain and loss of function. All possible fractures must be gently handled and carefully inspected. LOOK, FEEL and ASK the person if he can move the limb.

LOOK   There will be swelling and bruising, sometimes marked deformity. Is the skin intact? If not you are dealing with a potentially infected COMPOUND fracture.

FEEL   There will be tenderness over the injured area. Is the limb beyond still warm? If not there may be damage to blood vessels, indicating a pressing need for hospital transfer.

ASK   Can the injured person move the limb? This
            loss of function is typical. If you gently move
            the bone ends a *crunching* will be heard as they
            rub together. This is called CREPITUS. It is
            not necessary to demonstrate this. It produces
            pain but clinches the diagnosis — clinically.
X-RAY   This confirms the diagnosis. If you suspect a
            fracture, arrange hospital care AS SOON AS
            POSSIBLE.
SPLINT or   Only apply splints or strapping to those frac-
STRAP   tures which are causing severe discomfort.
            Refer to Chapters 17 and 18 for details. (See
            also 'Fractured jaw?' Chapter 14.)
REMEMBER   Do not give the injured person anything to
            eat or drink. Give reassurance and encourage-
            ment.

How To Stop Bleeding

Bleeding can occur from veins, in which case the blood is dark
in colour and flows out at a constant rate. It can also occur from
arteries.

Blood from arteries is bright red and squirts out in an inter-
mittent manner in time with the pulse.

Venous bleeding (bleeding from veins)

ELEVATE an injured limb.
APPLY pressure to the wound with gauze swabs. If the bleeding is on the face or body, firm pressure will control it.
BANDAGE the bleeding wound if possible, having first placed
a firm gauze pack upon it.

Arterial bleeding

APPLY firm pressure directly over the injured area for several
minutes.
BANDAGE the area after keeping it under firm pressure. If
bleeding recurs through the bandage, reapply pressure.

NECK INJURY?

The answer to this question should always be 'maybe' since you cannot be certain there is no neck injury after a man has been floored and remains unresponsive or complains of limb tingling or weakness afterwards. Use the five-man life technique only if no specialised stretcher is available and you will ensure the safety of your injured club members and colleagues (Chapter 15).

THIS IS A TRUE EMERGENCY. IMMEDIATE HOSPITAL TRANSFER MUST BE ARRANGED.

CARDIAC ARREST

Over-stimulation of the vagus nerve in either the neck or the chest is probably the commonest cause of cardiac arrest in combat. Although the heart may stop beating for a number of reasons, we believe that a simple description of the vagal nerve is useful.

In Latin vagus means 'wanderer'. The English words 'vagabond' and 'vagrant' derive from the Latin root. The vagus nerve lives up to its title well. It arises in the brain and is in fact two nerves (one on each side) but is generally spoken of in the singular form.

From the brain it passes down the neck where it lies vertically, like a plumb line, in the groove between two great vessels on each side of the neck — the internal jugular vein and the carotid artery. Although it has already given branches to various structures just as it leaves the brain, it gives off even more in the neck. Branches pass from the main trunk to the pharynx (the space behind the mouth and nasal passages), soft palate, trachea (gullet), and vocal cords. It even sends two special branches to the heart from the neck. Wandering into the chest it supplies important branches to the windpipe, lungs and heart. In this position it runs along the side of the gullet which it follows into the abdominal cavity. Here it stimulates the stomach, liver and pancreas. Leaving the stomach, the nerve travels on to supply all the small bowel and a sizeable part of the large bowel. It even sends branches along the arteries to the kidneys.

In the abdominal cavity the vagus is responsible for normal

functions of which we are unaware, such as acid production in the stomach and movement of the bowel muscles. In the chest its branches give sensation to the gullet, windpipe and lungs. Its influence on the heart is vital. Here it acts to keep the heart-beat slow and regular. Without the vagus nerve an important heart control mechanism would be lost.

Under normal circumstances the vagus will regulate heart rate. If, however, the nerve is suddenly abnormally stimulated from a punch to the chest or neck it will relay a message to the brain which reacts by 'shutting off everything'. This effectively slows the heart so much that it may stop beating. This is known as VAGAL CARDIAC ARREST. It occurs because the nerve is overstimulated. The heart will not recover unless immediate external cardiac massage is instituted.

One of the most famous historical examples of vagal cardiac inhibition is that of pregnant women who submitted themselves to the dubious skills of back-street abortionists. When the neck of the womb was stretched, nerve fibres were abnormally stimulated. These in turn relayed back to vagal fibres which responded by stopping the heart by reflex inhibition. This was a well-known occupational hazard for abortionists. Although their trade was in demand the disposal of dead bodies presented embarrassing interludes and taxed their ingenuity.

The course of the vagus nerve is illustrated opposite.

The unconscious fighter

A fighter may be unconscious for three reasons:
1. He may be knocked out. (see Chapter 11).
2. His heart may have stopped beating (CARDIAC ARREST).
3. He may have stopped breathing (RESPIRATORY ARREST).

In each of these situations the A B C of first-aid resuscitation should be carried out.

A = Airway. Is it open? If not, gently extend the neck to make it clear (see Fig. 16). Remove any dirt from the mouth. Clear away any vomit or blood.

B = Breathing. If the airway has been opened, is the person breathing through it? If not, you must breathe for him/her by beginning ARTIFICIAL RESPIRATION. The only satisfac-

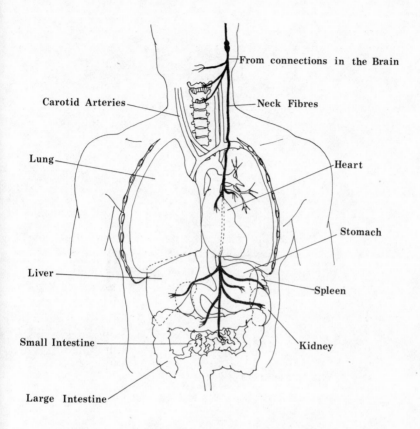

Fig. 15 The wanderings of the Vagus Nerve. The Vagus Nerve is especially vulnerable to abnormal stimulation from a blow to the neck or chest.

tory method is MOUTH-TO-MOUTH breathing. Watch the chest INFLATE as you breathe out. Do this every five or six seconds.

C = Circulation. Is there a carotid pulse in the neck? If not you must make it return by initiating EXTERNAL CARDIAC MASSAGE. This must be continued until EXPERT assistance is available.

B and C absent? This implies both cardiac and respiratory arrest. Therefore CARDIO-PULMONARY RESUSCITATION

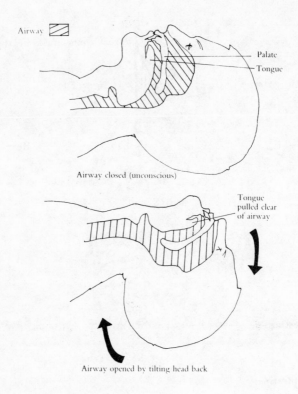

Fig. 16 How to open the airway in an unconscious person. Gently extend the neck.

must be started. Follow the instructions given below and the self-explanatory diagram (Fig. 17). Keep this process up until the patient recovers or EXPERT assistance becomes available.

REMEMBER THAT YOU SHOULD NOT THINK THAT YOU CAN PERFORM MOUTH-TO-MOUTH RESPIRATION AFTER READING THIS PAGE. YOU MUST ATTEND A FIRST-AID COURSE TO LEARN HOW TO GIVE ARTIFICIAL RESPIRATION OR DEAL WITH A CARDIAC ARREST.

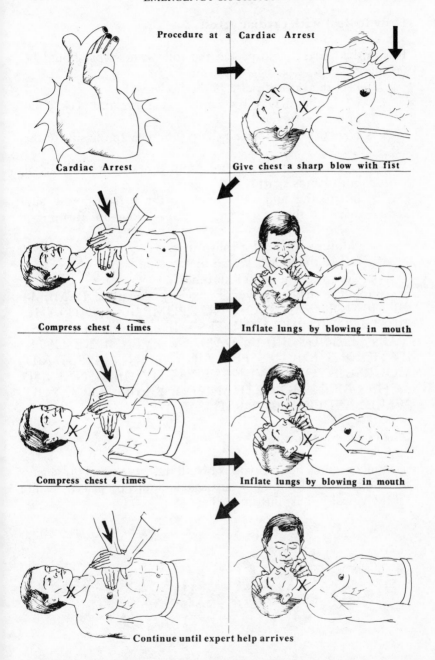

Fig. 17 The steps in heart–lung resuscitation.
X is the spot where the carotid pulse can be felt. Feel it in your own neck now.

How to deal with cardiac arrest

If a cardiac arrest is suspected the following steps should be taken:

1. Feel the carotid pulse in the neck.
2. Clear the airway by gently extending the neck if no pulse can be felt.
3. Give the breast bone a sharp thump with the side of the fist.
4. Compress the breast bone four times with the heels of both hands sharply.
5. Inflate the lungs by pinching the person's nose and exhaling firmly into his mouth — your lips forming a seal.
6. Compress the chest four times.
7. Inflate the lungs. Watch the chest inflate.
8. Compress the chest four times.

Continue until help arrives or recovery takes place. REMEMBER IF THE HEART DOES NOT PUMP BLOOD TO THE BRAIN FOR THREE MINUTES THE PERSON MAY SUSTAIN SERIOUS BRAIN DAMAGE EVEN IF RESUSCITATION IS SUCCESSFUL. ENROL IN A FIRST-AID COURSE IF YOU HAVE NEVER ATTENDED ONE OR IF IT HAS BEEN MORE THAN FIVE YEARS SINCE YOU WERE LAST ON A COURSE.

The coma position

The unconscious fighter who is breathing, has a good pulse and in whom no neck injury is suspected should be placed in the COMA position as illustrated (Fig. 18).

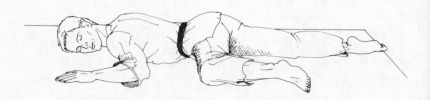

Fig. 18 The Coma position. Use it for the unconscious fighter who is breathing and in whom there is no suspicion of neck injury.

11.
HEAD INJURIES

'No head injury is too serious to be despaired of,
or too trivial to be ignored.'

Hippocrates

In most combat sports the head is a prime target. The successful
boxer can render his opponent unconscious with a punch; the
karateka can score ippon with a well-controlled kick or punch;
the wrestler or judoka can get a submission from a stranglehold
which affects the blood supply to the brain, thereby starving it
of oxygen. The head is a vulnerable area; the clever fighter uses
his, the poorer fighter loses his — and the fight.

ANATOMY OF THE HEAD

Have you ever wondered what brain tissue is like? It is so
delicate — rather like soft cheese — that during brain
operations the surgeon must be very careful not to apply
suction to it, otherwise it is simply sucked away. Because of its
vulnerability the brain is enclosed in a rigid bony box, the skull,
which acts like a big goldfish bowl. It is full of cerebro-spinal
fluid — CSF — which is produced in the brain and in which
the delicate brain itself floats. Among its many functions, CSF
acts as a cushion for the brain during movement of the head.
The brain is also covered with three membranes — a tough one
next to the skull, the others fine. In the spaces between these
membranes course blood vessels and CSF.

The brain itself has two main areas — the GREY MATTER
and the WHITE MATTER. GREY MATTER is the outside
part and is composed of millions of nerve cells. The WHITE
MATTER is the brain's core and is made up of the fibres which
come from the GREY MATTER. In the core there are, in
addition, specialised islands of GREY MATTER which have
different functions.

Remember that the GREY and WHITE MATTER are of
different consistencies — one is more dense or heavier than the
other.

WHY HEAD INJURIES ARE DIFFERENT

Head injuries are probably the most important injuries in sports. Unlike many other injuries they can be life-threatening, usually due to secondary complications rather than the severity of the initial impact. Many of the problems associated with these complications are preventable and the trainer must know what to do. In combat the chance of head injury is higher than in other sports. More important is the fact that if a fighter gets one head injury in a fight he has an even higher chance of getting another. The effects of this are discussed later.

WHAT HAPPENS IN A KNOCKOUT

When a fighter sustains a blow to the face or head, his head is accelerated backwards or jerked sidewards. Remember the brain is suspended in fluid inside the skull. The brain then moves the same way as the skull, only a split second or so later. Remember that the GREY and WHITE MATTER are of different consistencies. They get accelerated too, but at different rates. This causes the problem. The different rates lead to a SHEARING force between the GREY and WHITE MATTER. Some nerve cells are damaged, others die, never to be replaced. Depending on the strength of the blow, the fighter is knocked out for seconds or hours. What you must realise though is that some brain cells have died. Study Fig. 19. It summarises the effects of blows to the face and head upon the brain; you will note that the bi-directional arrows imply to-and-fro movement. The others imply collision of the brain with the skull. In a frontal blow both the front and the back of the brain can be damaged. This latter injury to brain tissue is called a CONTRE-COUP (opposite the blow) injury. It means that brain damage can occur at a distant site from the original punch. Obviously, many fighters get up, recover and can even win their bout, but the referee must be ever watchful of a man who has had a knock-out — even if he just went down and got back up.

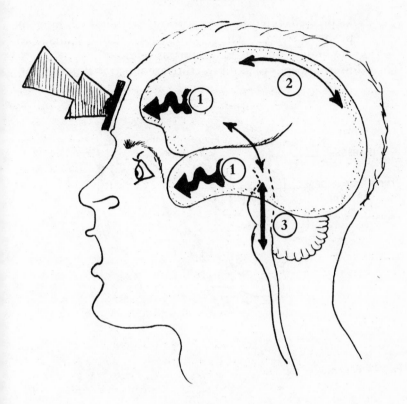

Fig. 19 The three-fold effects of a blow to the forehead.
(1) The direct effect at the front of the brain.
(2) The shearing effect at the opposite side of the brain from the impact. (This is sometimes called the contre coup effect.)
(3) The referred effect as the force of the blow is passed down the brain stem to the spinal cord.

FRACTURED SKULL

This means that one of the bones of the skull has been broken. It is important because it may either cause a blood clot which will then compress the brain, or it can lead to meningitis. For this reason alone doctors would keep a patient with a skull fracture, no matter how trivial, in hospital for twenty-four hours or more for observation.

Fractures can be of two types:
  1. Crack (linear) fractures running across the skull bones, which may tear the middle meningeal artery.

2. Depressed fractures. A portion of the skull bone is pushed inwards. The potential for causing damage to the brain from such an injury is obvious.

These differing types of skull fracture are illustrated in Fig. 20.

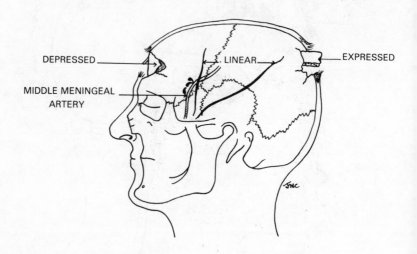

DEPRESSED

MIDDLE MENINGEAL
ARTERY

LINEAR

EXPRESSED

Fig. 20 Fractures of the skull.

BRAIN DAMAGE

The fighter who gets knocked out sustains some brain damage, although it is usually minor. Nerve cells have died and they never recover. Fortunately others take over their function, so the fighter appears normal. The damage done at this knock-out with loss of nerve cells is called PRIMARY damage. This damage can affect the whole brain and is known as DIFFUSE INJURY. When it affects only one part of the brain it is known as FOCAL INJURY.

We must now be careful to observe the fighter. Other things can happen. The membranes of the brain have blood vessels which can be torn and bleed, leading to pressure on the brain. (This can also happen if the skull is fractured.) There is a large artery running just under the skull which can be torn in a fracture. This too can lead to bleeding and pressure on the brain. When men have died after being knocked out in boxing, it is most often because of pressure on the brain caused by bleeding. This happens after the initial impact and is called SECONDARY damage. It is important to be aware of this since SECONDARY damage can be looked for and largely prevented.

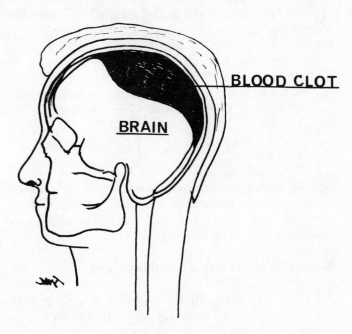

Fig. 21 A blood clot can compress the brain.

Results of primary brain damage

Primary brain damage can show itself in two ways:

1. *Concussion*

This term is not used much by doctors nowadays because it implies only temporary brain damage. Concussion is transient loss of consciousness — the knock-out. It is a diffuse type of damage. Return to normal is the rule within a few hours to a few weeks. However, doctors now know that any period of concussion is associated with death of some brain cells.

2. *Post-traumatic amnesia*

This term means loss of memory after a head injury — without necessarily being knocked out. The person can function apparently normally and automatically but remembers nothing afterwards. We can all remember footballers, rugby players and boxers who have been knocked out on the field, apparently recovered to finish the game, and then remember nothing about it afterwards.

Post-traumatic amnesia again implies diffuse primary brain damage with recovery the rule. To recognise it ask the following questions:
i)   Where are you?
ii)   Who are you?
iii) What hit you?
iv) What day, month, year is it?

If the person cannot answer these questions he should not continue, nor should any such fighter be allowed to fight or spar for a FOUR WEEK PERIOD.

Results of secondary brain damage

After primary brain injury, as we have said, secondary problems can set in and generally show themselves as progressive confusion or weakness in the limbs.

To avoid serious complications, these are indications for going to hospital:
1. Any fighter who is knocked out or has post-traumatic amnesia should be seen at hospital, where a decision will be made regarding skull X-ray.
2. If there is clear fluid from the nose or ear, this means there is a connection between the brain and the air and infection can set in.
3. If a fighter is knocked out, recovers and becomes drowsy or confused.
4. If one pupil gets bigger or smaller than the other and does not react to light by constricting.
5. If there is weakness or paralysis of any limb.
6. Any fighter who, despite regaining consciousness and remaining well orientated, complains of persistent

headache, vomits or feels generally unwell, should also be seen at hospital.

As a trainer you have a special responsibility where youngsters are involved. You, personally, should ensure their attendance at hospital, if required, and see them safely home. All hospital advice should be written down by you (most hospitals give head-injury instruction cards) and you should accurately relate both the events of the injury and the hospital advice to the child's parents. If hospital admission is required you should contact the parents and discuss the incident with them when they arrive.

Remember, head injuries can often appear trivial, especially when the injured person speaks sensibly afterwards. CAREFUL SUPERVISION IS NECESSARY FOR TWENTY-FOUR HOURS TO WATCH FOR SIGNS OF COMPLICATIONS (1-6 above).

Advice to wives and parents

Because a head injury may only become evident after several hours of normal consciousness and behaviour, it is essential to advise the wife or parents of a fighter to seek medical help *as soon as possible* if the person complains of double vision, headache or sickness, or if he becomes drowsy or confused.

If a fighter lives alone it is wise to check he is all right late in the evening after he has been unconscious, and again the next morning. NEVER DRINK ALCOHOL IN THE TWENTY-FOUR HOURS AFTER A HEAD INJURY. YOU SHOULD NOT DRIVE A CAR IF YOU HAVE BEEN UNCONSCIOUS.

THE IMPLICATIONS OF MINOR HEAD INJURIES

The primary head injuries we have discussed have in general been minor, with recovery the rule. We must appreciate however that if it is very severe, people can die of primary damage alone.

What happens if we test people psychologically in the four to six weeks after a minor head injury? Studies confirm that they have great difficulty in performing simple tests — adding, subtracting, etc. This does recover after four to six weeks but is a good reason why the Boxing Control bodies insist on a compulsory lay-off period after a knock-out. What happens if a person has had a second head injury during that six-week period? If the tests are repeated, the results are even poorer. Multiple minor head injuries therefore reduce the brain power and it can take up to three months or more for these mental processes to return to normal.

Post-traumatic syndrome

Sometimes after a knock-out the fighter gets headaches, dizziness, sleeplessness and is irritable. Work becomes difficult because concentration is poor. This is called the POST-TRAUMATIC or POST-CONCUSSIONAL SYNDROME. It can last for weeks to months or even longer. We think that this condition could be avoided in many people if injury to the head were given more respect.

Punch drunk syndrome

In the late 1930s when boxing was very popular, doctors began to notice that those who had been in the ring for years either as fighters or even just sparring partners developed slurring of the speech, a staggering gait and sometimes social incompetence. They appeared drunk — PUNCH DRUNK. Doctors now know that successive minor primary head injuries will lead to this condition. Since 1974, because control of fights has been stringent, there have been no cases in this country.

There is no place for being complacent. The condition could return through uncontrolled combat sports and the newer forms of karate, e.g. full contact, give cause for concern. This sport must comply with the same stringent rules as boxing.

You get the same thing in other sports — steeple-chase jockeys, rugby players, footballers and parachutists all suffer. It is totally irreversible. We all naturally lose brain cells but when this is compounded by a head injury it becomes noticeable as early as 35-45 years. Do you think that this is a justifiable risk?

PREVENTION OF HEAD INJURIES

We recently carried out a study on head injuries in sport (1980).

Surprisingly, we found that sports such as golf (when played by children), horse-riding and soccer had a higher incidence of serious head injuries than boxing or karate. The important point, though, is that in golf injuries can be easily dealt with by keeping children under supervision, by wearing protective head-gear in riding, and by encouraging the injured player to retire in soccer. The problem in our sport is the repeated minor injury. How do we prevent it?

We all agree that a knock-out can be easily sustained. Often the injured man falls backwards to strike his head on the floor. In boxing the ring floor is sprung and covered with canvas stretched over padding which is of a type and thickness approved by the Boxing Board of Control. Studies of head injuries in karate too have shown that padded flooring will prevent their number and severity. There are no specific regulations, but the Martial Arts Commission recommends that flooring should be of absorbent padding at least 1 cm thick and preferably of the interlocking type.

Another important area is headgear. When boxers spar they wear headgear which reduces injury. Why not wear it in competition? The reason is that the prospect of padded fighters would not appeal to the public. Perhaps this will take time.

Prevention of secondary brain damage

This depends on recognising the risks involved after certain types of injury already discussed, and ensuring that medical aid is sought. The trainer must know what to do.

Post-traumatic amnesia or a change in conscious level indicate brain injury. You should question such fighters carefully to detect disorientation or confusion. If a fighter has been unconscious, he should go to hospital for further examination since secondary complications are more likely. Also if there is confusion, double vision or weakness of an arm or leg, he should be seen in hospital. All scalp lacerations should be treated in hospital.

Prevention of cumulative damage

We discussed loss of brain cells from even a minor head injury which produces post-traumatic amnesia. The effects of repeated minor head injuries add up — i.e. they are CUMULATIVE.

The more we get the worse we end up until in extreme cases we are PUNCH DRUNK. This is why the governing bodies of boxing and steeple-chase have made rules regarding lay-off times after injury. They recommend a lay-off of four weeks after an episode of unconsciousness — no matter how brief.

Recent research suggests that it is not only combat sports that should be put under the microscope. Association football, rugby, climbing and even hockey should be aware of these injuries. Every year about 20,000 knock-outs occur in amateur sports of all types. The long-term results could be frightening if adequate measures for the prevention of further injury are not introduced.

RECOMMENDATIONS

We think that in all sport the following rules should be observed:

1. If the POST-TRAUMATIC condition is present — headaches, dizziness, poor concentration — NO SPORT until the symptoms have settled.
2. If there are three or more injuries leading to concussion or post-traumatic amnesia — NO FURTHER SPORT until examined by a specialist.
3. If there has been COMA — NO FURTHER COM-BAT SPORT. (Coma = a period of prolonged unconsciousness — more than one hour.)
4. Always have a doctor present at competitions.
5. Train and spar to improve your skills — not 'scar' your sparring partner.
6. Both the referee and the governing body must be stringent in their rules and decisions regarding these sports.

12.
INJURIES TO THE FACE

WHY FACIAL INJURIES ARE IMPORTANT

Our psychological and social well-being depends very much on how we appear. Unfortunately there are almost always stigmata to having a heavily scarred face. This fact aside, the fact is an important area. It has many vital structures, all of which are vulnerable to attack. Furthermore, there is great potential for injury prevention in this area.

ANATOMY OF THE FACE

The skeleton of the face maintains the shape of its soft tissues — the skin and muscles which overlie it. The forehead consists of the frontal bone of the skull; the middle part of the face contains the cheek and nasal bones. It also includes the upper jaw, teeth and lip. The lower part of the face comprises the lower jaw, teeth and lip. The lower jaw is an important structure, for in addition to its function in chewing it allows access to the airway and gullet. Sometimes in a severely broken jaw such access can be lost and difficulty experienced in ensuring that the tongue does not block the airway.

The muscles of the face assist in the acts of breathing, chewing and also facial expression.

The ear comprises the external ear and internal ear. The external ear is a cartilage flap covered by skin. It can be injured during punches or kicks and bleeding can occur. A late effect of this can be CAULIFLOWER EAR. The internal ear is a canal which runs inside the skull to the eardrum (tympanic membrane). It is a very fine membrane stretched across the ear canal. Attached to it on its inside are several small bones which transform the energy of the vibrating drum into waves which our brains interpret as comprehensible sounds. This innermost part of the ear has a further important function: that of balance. So when its function is impaired one of the symptoms may be dizziness (vertigo).

The nose is the first-line organ for the sense of smell and the function of breathing. Obviously, any injury could make breathing more difficult.

TYPES OF FACIAL INJURY

Lacerations and abrasions

These are probably the commonest injuries in combat sport. Almost every boxer after a hard exchange will have reddening of the skin around the cheeks and eye sockets. If the skin is broken he may have only an abrasion — a graze. This requires simple washing with a disinfectant solution (Dettol).

Cuts (lacerations), however, are more important because they can stop the fight or if treated poorly leave a weak area of scar tissue which will bleed again in a subsequent fight. The fighter now has a 'cut' problem. Recurrent cuts also eventually produce unsightly scars.

Treatment of cuts during the contest must be within the limits of the rules. We would advise that, unless absolutely necessary, cut areas should not be allowed to be subject to further punishment.

Emergency treatment

The cut should first be carefully inspected, during a round if necessary. It is then up to the seconds, between rounds, to ensure that bleeding stops. This can be achieved by permissible styptic materials followed by the light application of grease. This will minimise any further damage. If the cut is serious enough to cause stoppage it should then be sutured (sewn up) by an experienced doctor who is well aware of the problems associated with combat sport. These are not cuts for the inexperienced. Boxing promoters would do well to ensure that the services of a surgeon were at least on hand to deal with such emergencies.

Special areas

Cuts around the eye are especially troublesome. Those above the eye can impair vision and so endanger the fighter. Those below the eye tend to gape more but generally do not impair vision. The face is well supplied with blood so heavy bleeding is common, especially on the forehead or lips. Examine them carefully. Keep the fighter's safety in mind. If there is any doubt ask the doctor.

Prevention

Everything possible should be done during training or sparring to prevent cuts. Headgear should be worn. The avoidance of head clashing in the fight itself is an important aim. Fighters who persistently butt put their opponent at risk and should be penalised.

How to treat a bleeding nose

In most sports except boxing a bleeding nose would lead to a competition being stopped. The effective method of management is to sit the person erect and get him to pinch his nose between thumb and index finger with a swab or handkerchief (tissue is satisfactory). Bleeding will stop in about five to six minutes in most cases. If it continues or is particularly severe this may imply more extensive injury. The patient should be taken to an accident and emergency department for treatment. Transport is possible with the injured man sitting up pinching his nose. Other methods such as instructing the patient to lie flat result in him swallowing blood which causes nausea and vomiting. Ice or keys dropped down the back may be an effective method in folk-lore but in practice they are unsuccessful.

Injuries to the lips

Many cuts to the lips can be prevented by wearing a gumshield. This should ideally be designed by your dentist, but failing this the malleable type, which is moulded to the contours of the mouth after immersion in warm water, is better than no protection. Most lip injuries bleed profusely but heal well. If there is a gaping cut, sutures (stitching) may be required. Remember to inspect for broken teeth. Tooth fragments can also become embedded in the lips producing delay in healing. If there is a broken tooth and cut lip, the wound should be inspected by the doctor.

Injuries to the ears

Injuries to the external ear occur especially in boxing and wrestling. These take the form of lacerations or frequent bleeding underneath the skin, producing a large bruise. The ear then has a bluish, swollen appearance and is hot and tender to touch. If this is left alone it will lead to disfigurement of the ear — the CAULIFLOWER EAR — with thickening and distortion. Imediate treatment is with ice packing, but all such injuries should be seen by the club doctor as soon as possible. He will be able to disperse the swelling with specific preparations.

BONY INJURIES

Broken nose?

The most common nasal injury following a hard blow is a fracture or mobilising of the nasal bones. This may occur with or without deformity of the nose. The injury may be compound (when the bones protrude through the skin) or simple (when only the bones are broken with no break in the skin).

If the injury is inspected at the time it happens and before marked swelling has occurred, it can be reduced immediately. The bones are firmly moulded with finger pressure so that the nose appears straight. If this is not immediately successful it should be abandoned.

Hospital inspection is always recommended even if the injury is a week old or more. The nasal bones can be manipulated up to almost three weeks after injury.

In boxing, recurrent nasal injury eventually produces the classical picture of the 'Boxer's Nose'. If this produces difficulty with breathing or is cosmetically unacceptable corrective treatment should be delayed until the individual has retired. from combat sports.

Broken cheek-bone

The cheek-bone can be felt just in front of the ear. It passes across the face to the nose and can be felt with the finger throughout its length. It gives the middle part of the face its fullness.

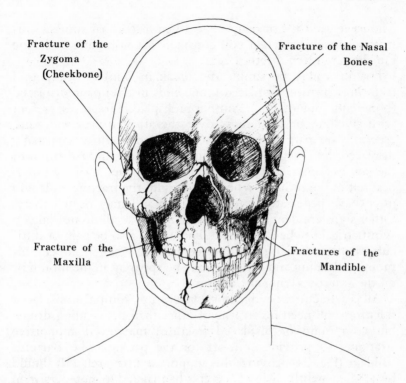

Fracture of the
Zygoma
(Cheekbone)

Fracture of the Nasal
Bones

Fracture of the
Maxilla

Fractures of the
Mandible

Fig. 22 Fractures of the facial bones.

Fractures result from direct blows and produce characteristic signs. Usually the bone is depressed — that is, pushed inwards — so the face is asymmetrical and flattened. There is also an obvious depression on the affected side. Several other important diagnostic signs exist. There is difficulty in opening the mouth. Often the person talks through his teeth. If you touch the skin on the affected cheek there may be numbness. This is because a nerve which gives sensation to the skin of the face has been injured in the fracture.

Broken cheek-bones need surgical attention to correct the deformity and transfer to hospital is necessary.

Broken jaw?

The lower jaw is not comonly broken in combat sports. This may surprise you when you consider that in boxing or karate punches are often directed at it.

Fractures may be simple (no break in skin) or compound (skin broken too), displaced (bone ends in line) or undisplaced (bone ends out of line). Simple undisplaced fractures present with swelling or tenderness over the affected area and pain, especially on gritting the teeth. Compound fractures are usually displaced. Swelling and deformity are present and palpation of the jaw as shown in Fig. 23 may reveal a gap. Usually this is best felt in the mouth. When compound, the fracture ends will often have penetrated into the mouth and may be felt there. Other signs are dental malocclusion — the teeth do not line up symmetrically when clenched. There may also be pain or difficulty experienced by the injured person when he opens his mouth. Bleeding and bruising may be apparent in the mouth or on the skin overlying the fracture.

All jaw fractures need medical inspection. Simple undisplaced fractures will need no treatment other than pain-killing drugs, but compound or displaced fractures may need supportive strapping to provide comfort for the patient. The Barton's bandage (Fig. 24) provides this support and pain relief. It should be applied gently using 2″ crepe bandage. Do not persist in applying it if the injured person complains of intolerable pain or feelings of sickness.

ALL COMPOUND FRACTURES NEED HOSPITAL TREATMENT. DO NOT GIVE THE INJURED PERSON ANYTHING TO EAT OR DRINK SINCE THE TREATMENT MAY INVOLVE AN OPERATION.

Whenever a facial fracture involving the nose, jaw or cheek has occurred, a lay-off of between six to twelve weeks will be required. The injured person should be examined medically before *fighting* again. Training may resume earlier but contact should not be allowed.

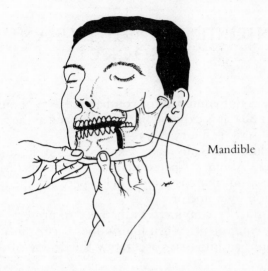

Mandible

Fig. 23 Gentle examination of a suspected fracture for movement. This should only be done by those who have attended First Aid courses.

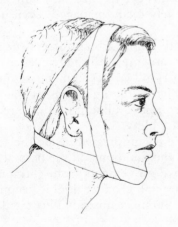

Fig. 24 Barton's Bandage (to support suspected fractures of the jaw).

13.
INJURIES TO THE EYE AND EYE SOCKET

The eye is not equipped for combat. It has no bony shell, only two soft lids. It is exposed both in front and at the side. It is vital and any serious injury is tragic.

Eye injuries, sadly, are very common in all sports and pastimes. About 90 per cent are preventable. Many lead to blindness, but there is often a delay between the injury and its evaluation by a doctor.

You must be convinced of the need to protect yourself with suitable equipment. When injury does occur the aim is to preserve sight and to assess accurately the degree of damage.

TYPES OF EYE INJURY

Foreign bodies such as dust, dirt or splinters can enter the eye and irritate its coverings, producing conjunctivitis or a tear in the outer covering of the eye (corneal abrasion). Such problems are minor and relatively easily managed, even if the particle is embedded.

If the eye is compressed by a blunt object such as the heel or fist, very large forces are imparted to the eyeball and its internal structures. This can result in detachment of the retina at the back of the eye, which is the light-sensitive area. Its loss can produce partial or complete blindness. Rupture of the eyeball can also follow such a blow.

Sometimes the eye is compressed inside the socket but does not rupture. Instead the thin bones at the base of the eye socket burst. Paralysis of eye movements from entrapment of ocular muscles in the fracture will produce double vision. This is called a blow-out fracture. Its mechanism is illustrated in Fig. 25.

Head injuries and impairment of vision

An injury to almost any part of the head can produce visual

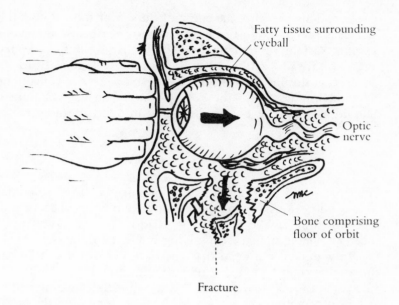

Fig. 25 Blow-out fracture of the eye socket.

symptoms, often temporary. If a person has sustained an obvious head injury and complains of blurred or double vision, this is an indication that hospital care is needed.

Black eyes

This is a bruise of the eye socket and lids. The colour and swelling are caused by bleeding into the skin. Every black eye should be seen by a doctor to allow exclusion of serious eye injury or skull fracture.

Lacerations around the eye socket can cause considerable bleeding and can even stop the fight. Inspect both the laceration and the eye before making the decision that the fighter can continue.

PROTECTIVE DEVICES

The theory behind eye protection is that the stronger frontal bones and cheek-bones should allow diffusion of the forces. Therefore a head guard should be prominent above and below the eye. This prevents the entry of the fist or foot. Remember that it is preferable to receive a cut above or below the eye or even to sustain a fractured cheek-bone than serious eye injury. Fig. 3 illustrates a type of head guard which can afford eye protection during sparring. Find one and wear one. Encourage your colleagues to do the same. Boxers and contact fighters should have regular examinations by an ophthalmologist.

THE ONE-EYED FIGHTER

This presents a dilemma for the sports organisation. In boxing one-eyed persons are not allowed to take part, but karate, judo and wrestling make no such legislation. There have already been avoidable tragedies involving one-eyed fighters.

We would recommend that one-eyed persons may take part in combat training but that no sparring should be permitted. If the person is insistent on combat, the guidelines would be that after informative discussion with a doctor, officials in the governing body and possibly even a solicitor, appropriate waivers be signed. All sparring should take place wearing protection approved by the medical control body of the sport.

FIRST AID

First-aid equipment for eye injuries

Phone numbers of the nearest hospitals, especially eye hospitals with a casualty service, should be at hand in all clubs. This is extremely important as not all hospitals may have an eye surgeon on call. It is your responsibility as a trainer/coach to find out what services are available in your locality. This is easily done by contacting the Health Authority Board or administration offices.

A vision card, penlight and protective eye cover make up part of the equipment. In addition, tapes, cotton swabs (sterile) and sterile irrigation solutions should be acquired. All further necessary treatment can be performed by the doctor.

Examination of eye injuries

Remember that serious eye injury is not always immediately apparent. Examine the injured eye carefully. Check that the person can see the vision card. Use the penlight to examine the iris (the coloured part) and pupil. If they are uneven or you can see blood behind the pupil, assume the injury is serious. Double vision and unequal eye movements imply damage. Arrange hospital referral. If you are unable to open the eye because of swelling do not force the lids apart, since if the ball of the eye is ruptured you may squeeze its contents out. Be content to apply a patch gently over the eye and tape it into position without pressing it too hard on the eye. Tell the victim not to apply pressure to the eye either.

Remember you are trying to ascertain whether or not an injury has occurred. If in doubt do not let the fighter continue and get expert help.

First aid for minor injuries

Foreign body in the eye

Advise the person to blink the eye two or three times rapidly. This may remove the foreign body. Do not let him rub the eye as this will make the condition worse. Gently pull the upper lid so that it overlaps the lower lid. This too may allow removal of the foreign body.

If these are unsuccessful, seat the injured person in a good light and ask him to look up, to the right, left, down and along his nose. You should stand behind him with a sterile cotton wool swab or the edge of a clean handkerchief. Any foreign body seen should be gently wiped off. If it does not come off it may have penetrated the eye. Cover the eye with a pad and take the person to hospital.

Irrigation with sterile saline is another method of dislodgement which is often effective.

ALL OTHER EYE INJURIES SHOULD BE SEEN BY A DOCTOR.

14.
INJURIES TO THE TEETH AND JAW

Dental injuries are rarely regarded as serious. This is a paradox because of all tissues in the body the teeth have least ability for self repair. Once injured, the natural process is towards further decay and damage. Dental injury produces discomfort and social embarrassment and treatment can be expensive. Prevention is cheap and effective but boxing is the only sport where this principle is effectively applied.

TYPES OF DENTAL INJURY

The teeth consist of an outer part, the crown covered with enamel, and a root embedded in the bone of the jaw. Within the enamel is dentine and the tooth pulp which lies in the centre. It contains the nerves and blood vessels. Surrounding the root in the gum is a fine membrane that fixes the tooth in its socket. (See Fig. 26.)

Following a blow the crown may break or crack, the root may be broken, the tooth can be dislocated backwards, forwards or even driven into the bone like a nail into wood.

Complications

We noted that decay can occur after dental fracture. However, even if a tooth sustains a mild blow — not enough to cause a fracture — the pulp may be damaged and the tooth may 'die' within a few weeks. Such a tooth will require root treatment to maintain its health. A final problem with chipped or broken teeth is that the fragments can become embedded in the lips. If this is not recognised infection will follow, delaying healing of the lip laceration.

First-aid treatment

With a chipped or broken tooth a fighter should be advised to stop, since further blows to the face will almost certainly cause

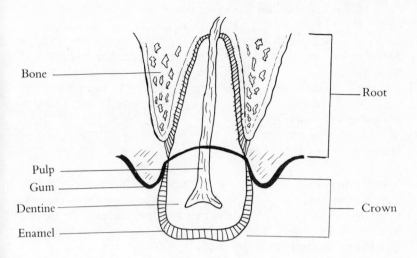

Fig. 26 Anatomy of a tooth. Teeth have no capacity for repair.

bleeding. He should keep his mouth closed to prevent exposure of the sensitive exposed dentine to the air.

If dental dislocation occurs, realignment must be attempted immediately. Even if the tooth is completely dislodged it should be washed and quickly pushed back into its socket. If it is left out of the mouth for longer than half an hour the chances of it surviving are minimal. Once this has been done, take the patient to a dentist.

If there are cuts about the mouth, local pressure with gauze swabs either inside or outside will control bleeding until they can be carefully examined by a doctor.

FRACTURED JAW?

The lower jaw is most commonly broken from punches to the face. The upper jaw rarely sustains such an injury. The early recognition of this injury is easy if the mouth is hanging open, if there is marked swelling and deformity of the jaw or bleeding inside the mouth where the broken fragments have torn the gums. Much more difficult to recognise are the breaks with no displacement of the fragments. Ask the injured man to open and close his mouth. He should be able to do this opposing his teeth accurately. If he winces or you succeed in producing pain along the jaw by gently feeling it, assume he has a fracture. Transfer to hospital is required.

How to strap a bad break

A badly broken jaw is usually attended by concussion. Therefore, the victim needs to be seen at hospital on both counts. When there is severe deformity, gently apply a supporting crepe bandage of the type illustrated in Fig. 24 to relieve pain until a detailed examination can be made.

MOUTH PROTECTION

Boxing, for once, is not the offending sport! Coaches and participants have known for years the protective effect of gumshields. Not only do they splint the teeth but they also protect against knock-outs. Mouth guards have been shown in laboratory studies to reduce the frequency of this injury.

Probably traditional karate is the worst offender. Although contact to the face is forbidden, mouth injuries occur in about 10-15% of all contests. Injuries to the teeth complicate half of these. When we consider that there are several thousand karate bouts in a year this adds up to a large number of broken teeth!

Types of guard

The most frequent criticism of guards is that they don't stay in place. Most are bought from the sports shop. Although these are adequate we suggest you have one (or two) made by your dentist. They fit snugly and after a few sessions you won't feel uncomfortable. They do not fall out when the mouth is opened. Wrestling and judo can also be practised wearing a shield, although dental injury is less common in these sports.

RECOMMENDATIONS

Dental injuries are almost 100% preventable. We recommend custom-built gum-shields to protect the teeth and jaws and reduce the frequency of knock-out.

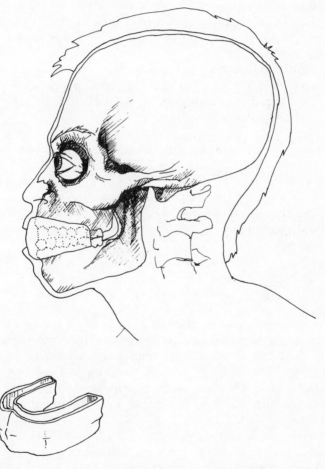

Fig. 27 Wear a gum shield. It protects the teeth, the bones of the face and reduces the chance of being knocked out.

15.
INJURIES TO THE NECK AND BACK

Injuries to the bones of the spine, especially to the neck, can be the most devastating of all. Neck injuries occur because:
1. The head is accelerated by a kick or punch.
2. The neck is compressed and twisted as in landing badly after a throw.
3. Rotation of the neck occurs when the head is fixed and flexed as in landing badly in judo, or over-extending as in illegally breaking the wrestler's bridge by jumping on one's opponent.

Although neck injuries are uncommon they can produce DEATH or PARALYSIS. Therefore PREVENTION is paramount. If injury does occur, injudicious first-aid measures may WORSEN a treatable injury. You cannot learn how to care for such injuries from a book. Only by attendance at organised first-aid courses run by qualified persons can such knowledge be acquired.

ANATOMY OF THE NECK AND BACK

Look at the diagram of the spinal column. It consists of small bones strung together like cotton reels. These bones are called VERTEBRAE and they are bound to each other by ligaments and joints. These allow twisting, turning and bending movements to be performed under the influence of the powerful muscles which support the spine and provide strength and mobility.

The vertebrae in the neck are called CERVICAL vertebrae. There are seven of them. They are followed by twelve THORACIC vertebrae (supporting the ribs), five LUMBAR, FIVE SACRAL and a variable number of COCCYGEAL (tail bone) vertebrae.

Each vertebra consists of a body and an arch. The body is sturdy and supports the body weight at each level. The arch protects the spinal cord which is a solid flex of nervous tissue

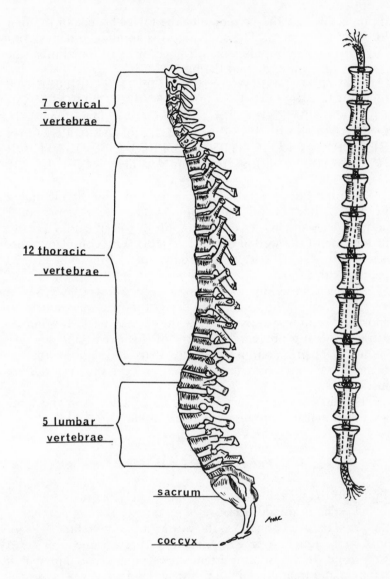

7 cervical
vertebrae

12 thoracic
vertebrae

5 lumbar
vertebrae

sacrum

coccyx

Fig. 28 The spinal column (side view). The bones are held together by ligaments and small joints. The spinal cord runs through a tunnel formed by the vertebrae similar to cotton reels threaded together.

running through the vertebrae to the lower border of the first LUMBAR vertebra. The spinal cord is about as thick as your finger. It carries impulses from the brain to all four limbs, the muscles of respiration and the heart.

IF SEVERE DISPLACEMENT OF THE VERTEBRAE OCCURS BECAUSE ONE IS FRACTURED OR BECAUSE ONE BECOMES DISLOCATED FROM THE ONE ABOVE OR BELOW IT, THE SPINAL CORD CAN BE TORN ACROSS. THIS WILL PRODUCE DEATH OR PARALYSIS DEPENDING ON THE LEVEL OF DAMAGE.

The importance of the level of injury is graphically illustrated in the method of judicial hanging. The tailor-made collar ensures extreme hyper-extension of the neck and fracture-dislocation of the second cervical vertebra with complete trans-ection of the spinal cord at this point. Such an injury is incompatible with life.

However, let us suppose the injury is at a lower level, say at vertebra five, six or seven. This type of injury can result from sport and produce paralysis below the chest or neck. It is indeed a tragedy that a preventable injury of this extent and severity should happen. You must ensure that all methods recommended by your governing body to prevent such injuries are instituted.

The possible effects of injuries at various levels in the spine are illustrated in diagrammatic form in Fig. 30.

PREVENTION OF INJURY

Injury to the neck bones are the most likely because:
    1. The head and neck are often targets.
    2. The neck bones are the most mobile vertebrae.
It is therefore of extreme importance to prevent the injury ever occurring. It is also important to recognise the injury if it happens and treat it safely until medical aid arrives. The principles of prevention are:
    1. Prevention through fitness
    2. Prevention through skill
    3. Prevention of illegal moves
    4. Prevention through first-aid training.

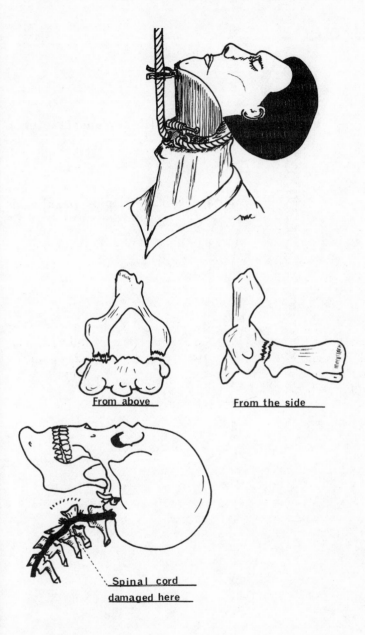

From above

From the side

Spinal cord
damaged here

Fig. 29 The Hangman's Fracture. Fracture of the arch of the second cervical vertebra :C2) leads to complete division of the spinal cord. At this level of division survival is impossible.

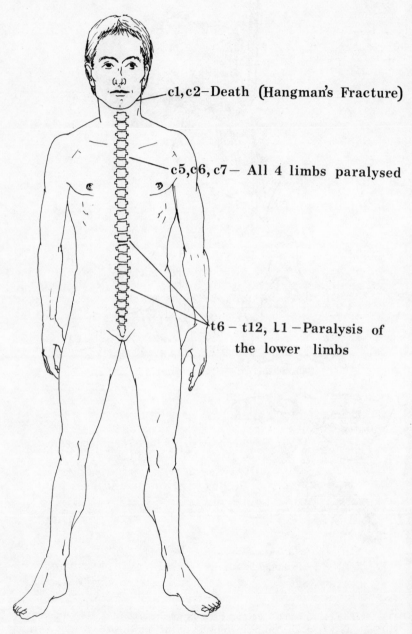

c1,c2–Death (Hangman's Fracture)

c5,c6,c7– All 4 limbs paralysed

t6 – t12, L1 –Paralysis of
the lower limbs

Fig. 30 Effects of severe damage to the spinal cord at different levels.

Prevention through fitness

All training programmes should include exercises which will
increase the suppleness of the neck. The best are those in which
the fighter moves his neck forward until his chin drops on his
chest, backwards until his chin is pointing in the air, and finally
turns the head from side to side. Try this last exercise now. Try
to turn your chin until it is pointing directly over one shoulder,
then try to turn your head just a little bit further very slowly
and gently.

The strength of neck muscles can be increased by isometric
exercises, that is by trying to move the head against the
resistance of your own hand. Try this now. Turn your head
halfway towards one shoulder, then try to push it back
to mid-line using the hand on the side to which the head is
pointing.

It takes a little time to achieve the correct balance between
arm and neck muscles but you will soon find that you can make
your neck muscles work hard by using the resistance of other
muscles.

Isotonic exercises, that is those in which the neck muscles are
in movement while acting against an external force, are also
very important. A simple head harness allows the use of
weights over the neck muscles which can then be given weight
training.

Extreme power can be generated in the neck muscles. The
wrestler especially protects his neck muscles and their potential
is demonstrated by his ability to do 'bridge-presses' with very
heavy weights. You should not attempt this though until you
have performed basic strengthening exercises.

Prevention through skill

All grappling sports should give specific advice on how to avoid
neck injury by correct falling techniques. Escape from strangleholds should be skilfully executed without putting the neck at
risk. Boxers and karatekae of all styles should practise the skills
of 'riding' and 'slipping' punches or kicks. Finally, fair weight
matching and equivalent experience of fighters prevent injury.

Prevention of illegal moves

Rabbit punching and chops to the side of the neck are forbidden. Because of their potential seriousness we would advise the governing bodies to take a stern view of fighters who use these techniques.

Rotational kicks such as the spinning back kick are also dangerous and should be excluded from competition. The technique of KAKATO (high heel stamp kick) can produce both serious head injury and hyper-extension neck injury. We recommend that this technique should also be made illegal.

Certain judo throws involve risk to the neck and should not be attempted by beginners impressed by experts demonstrating them.

In the wrestling bridge an opponent should not collapse the bridge by direct pressure. This method was the cause of many deaths in Russia until the rules were altered. The correct method is to attempt to flex your opponent's neck by pulling his head forwards.

Prevention through first-aid training

We do not intend to try to include a description of the safest means of giving first-aid treatment to someone who has had a neck injury or who is in need of mouth-to-mouth resuscitation. We believe that this *must be learned under the direct supervision of a skilled teacher*. The best approach is to enrol in a first-aid course and to encourage your own clubs and associations to develop seminars and coaching sessions on the prevention and treatment of injury.

INJURIES TO THE SPINE — NECK INJURIES

Serious injuries

Recognition

Serious neck injury should always be suspected:
1. If a fighter is lying unconscious on the floor after a throw, heavy kick or punch to the head or twisting headlock, possibly with his head at an unusual angle to his neck.

2. If a fighter is conscious but says he cannot move his arms or legs or that he has pins and needles in his arms, even if he does not complain of pain in the neck.
3. If a fighter who is able to move his arms and legs complains of pain in the neck after a blow, bad breakfall or twisting-lock.

Treatment

This is an extremely difficult subject. Each case is unique and incorrect treatment can make the damage worse. The first step is to ensure that the fighter can breathe properly. This is of vital importance and attendance at a course run by a qualified person is the best way of learning how to clear and keep clear the airway of an unconscious person. Once you are satisfied that the player can breathe, send for an ambulance and a doctor. Tell the ambulance station the nature of the injury you suspect and ask if they will bring a doctor from hospital if it is not possible to contact a doctor directly. DO NOT ATTEMPT TO MOVE THE FIGHTER UNTIL THE AMBULANCE ARRIVES. THE COMPETITION SHOULD BE STOPPED UNTIL IT DOES.

MOVING A PERSON WITH A NECK INJURY REQUIRES THE USE OF SPECIAL STRETCHERS SKIL-FULLY PLACED. IF THESE ARE UNAVAILABLE A FIVE-MAN LIFT MAY BE REQUIRED. ONLY SKILLED PERSONNEL OR TRAINED FIRST-AIDERS SHOULD BE INVOLVED. This is another good reason why first-aid training is so important.

Less serious neck injuries

If the fighter has normal feeling in his limbs and can move them with no tingling, he probably has a muscle or ligament injury. He should stop fighting and ice should be applied to the injured area. If pain continues he should be seen at hospital as soon as possible as he may have a partial dislocation. If the pain abates within fifteen minutes he should be asked to move his neck gently and slowly. If movement is limited, he should be taken to hospital as soon as possible. If there is a full range of move-ment, the injury probably only affects muscles and ligaments and the fighter should continue to keep the area cool for

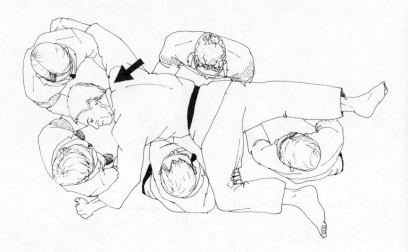

Fig. 31 If it becomes ABSOLUTELY NECESSARY to lift someone with a suspected neck injury, get the assistance of at least four others. Two will support the head and neck, two the trunk and pelvis, and one the legs.

twenty-four hours but he should try to keep it as mobile as possible.

Arteries, nerves and veins of the neck

Apart from the bones, other important structures are the trachea and oesophagus, the jugular veins, carotid arteries and vagus and phrenic nerves. In strangulation the carotid arteries may be compressed leading to unconsciousness within minutes because the brain is starved of blood. Chokes, on the other hand, will lead to compression of the windpipe. You will also recall how vulnerable the vagus nerve is.

Unconsciousness from strangles should be managed as if the person has had a head injury. Vagus nerve injury is also detailed elsewhere (Fig. 15).

Laryngeal injury

The larynx (voice box) is especially vulnerable in neck locks, chokes and strangles. Direct blows happen accidentally in karate and boxing.

Recognition

If the man has difficulty breathing he should immediately be taken to hospital. If an ice-pack is gently placed on the voice box and the fighter is kept upright this will help prevent swelling of the area.

Returning to train and fight

If medical advice has been obtained that training and competing can recommence the fighter should do so, provided he has no pain on swallowing and can talk or shout without discomfort.

BACK INJURIES

Injuries to the muscles, ligaments and vertebrae can occur in the grappling sports but are less common in punching and kicking sports. Minor injuries outnumber all others and consist mainly of muscular strains. These produce back pain and stiffness and are amenable to the ICE regime.

Back pain which produces persistent stiffness over a period of days or weeks, is unrelieved by rest, or is associated with burning or tingling feelings in the legs, requires investigation by a doctor. If you get such symptoms arrange to see your own doctor.

Returning to fight after neck or back injury

This will depend very much on the severity of the injury and the final result after treatment. If it was necessary to attend hospital for treatment, the advice of the doctor managing your case must be taken.

If the injury did not require attendance at hospital, training can restart when neck movements are full and pain-free. Actual combat must be postponed until you have reached your pre-injury fitness and can perform exercises normally.

16.
INJURIES TO THE CHEST AND ABDOMEN

The chest and abdomen (collectively the trunk) present a large target for attack and it is well known amongst boxers that effective body punching can weaken an opponent. A powerful technique to the chest or abdomen will be awarded with a score in karate. Amongst wrestlers and judoka the trunk may sustain accidental injury through falls or the application of pressure. The two regions are considered in turn.

ANATOMY OF THE CHEST

The chest or thorax lies between the neck and abdomen. It contains the heart and lungs, great vessels, gullet and the wind-pipe (trachea) with its divisions into bronchi. Each side of the chest wall consists of twelve ribs attached in front to the breast bone (sternum) and at the back to the thoracic vertebrae. The design of the ribs and their muscular attachments are such that the chest wall moves in and out like bellows as the individual breathes. The front of the chest is covered with the large pectoral muscles at the front and the large back muscles behind. These muscles are illustrated in Fig. 33. The shoulder blades are also attached to the back of the chest by large muscles. The shape of these bones and their joints to the upper arm allow an extensive range of movement of the limbs.

The ribs are for breathing. They also provide a little protection for the chest contents, but they are designed mainly for the movements of breathing. They are incapable of withstanding major crushing forces and when broken can occasionally penetrate the lungs and rupture them.

Within the chest, on either side, lie the lungs. They are two sponge-like structures containing millions of little spaces where oxygen diffuses into the blood. They are covered with a double membrane called the pleura. If the outer layer is burst from a penetrating injury the result is a ruptured lung.

The heart is the next important structure. It is divided into

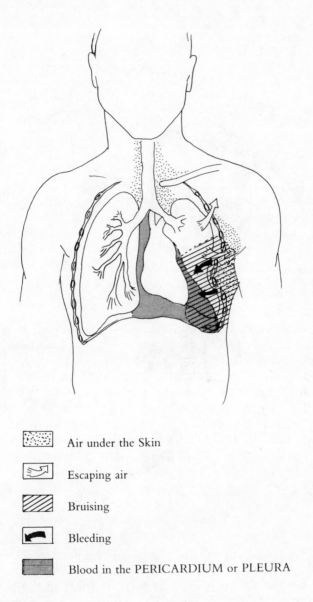

::::::	Air under the Skin
⤵	Escaping air
⁄⁄⁄	Bruising
◄	Bleeding
▬	Blood in the PERICARDIUM or PLEURA

Fig. 32 The effects of violence upon the chest.

four chambers, two of which deal with venous blood (blood
from the veins), receiving it and sending it through the lungs to

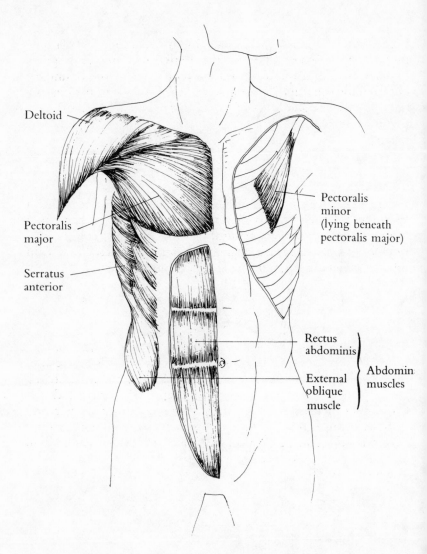

Fig. 33 The muscles of the chest and abdominal wall.

have oxygen added to it. It is then returned to the heart and received into the third chamber. From here it is pumped into the fourth chamber and into the body by means of the aorta, the largest artery in the body. It gives off branches to the head, neck, chest and back, and subsequently to the abdomen and legs.

The vagus nerve also runs in the chest where it sends branches to the lungs and heart. One other important nerve is present in the chest. This is the PHRENIC nerve. It gives branches to the diaphragm muscle which forms the boundary between the chest and abdominal cavity. Damage to the phrenic nerve causes problems with diaphragmatic movements and therefore breathing.

INJURIES TO THE SKIN

Lacerations, bruising and abrasions are especially common in those sports such as boxing and karate where the chest is a target. They can be very painful because the chest moves continually. Apply the basic principles already discussed. If pain relief is adequate, training need not be interrupted.

INJURIES TO MUSCLE

The pectoral muscles, being the largest of the chest wall, are most likely to be injured. You can feel them on the chest wall but also where they join the upper arm. Press your outstretched hand against the wall and feel your armpit. The firm band that runs along the front of the armpit is the tendon of the pectoral muscle. If this is torn because of a punch or kick it may require surgical treatment. Bear this in mind, for poor healing will almost certainly affect muscle power.

Bruising of the muscles between the ribs or over the back can also occur. ICE and aspirin in the early stages will control pain and swelling and provide a basis for adequate healing.

Breast injuries

The popularity of free fighting for women in judo and karate has meant that injuries to the breasts are seen more often than previously. The fatty tissue of the breast can become hard and tender after being punched. Bruising usually spreads to involve the lower breast and will settle in several days. Such injuries can be prevented by wearing a protective, firm-cup brassière. However, every breast lump should be inspected by a doctor even though you may be able to relate it to a punch or kick.

INJURIES TO BONE

Bruised or broken ribs are extremely disabling. Every time you cough your chest aches. Breathing becomes painful but pain relief with aspirin and support with your own hand when you cough will allow recovery. After bruised or broken ribs a lay-off of 10–21 days is required.

If a broken rib punctures a lung the problem is more serious. The ruptured lung collapses. Breathing becomes laboured and painful. Fortunately only one side is commonly involved. The person will have one good lung functioning, so your immediate action should be to keep him sitting up and transfer him to hospital immediately.

INJURIES TO THE CONTENTS OF THE CHEST

1. **Ruptured lung?**

Sudden breathlessness accompanied by chest pain after a blow should arouse suspicion. Often the injured man will become faint and sweat. He may even cough up a little blood. Let him sit erect or semi-erect and arrange hospital transfer.

Treatment In hospital a chest X-ray will confirm the diagnosis. Depending on its extent, further treatment in the form of a simple chest drain may be required. This will allow the lung to re-inflate.

2. **Blows to the heart**

Any blow to the centre or left side of the chest can affect the heart. In most instances nothing happens, but the vagus nerve can be overstimulated and lead to undue slowing or cardiac arrest. Adhere strictly to the ABC of first-aid (see Emergencies p. 90). External massage may be necessary. Keep it up until professional help is available.

PREVENTION OF CHEST INJURIES

The chest is amazingly well protected during fights. This seems to be a natural reaction. However, padded body armour can still be used to good effect. We would suggest that where there is a lot of bodily contact such protective clothes should be worn. Women should always wear well-fitting, padded or plastic cup brassières.

ANATOMY OF THE ABDOMEN

The abdominal cavity is the largest of the body cavities and is even more extensive than is at first apparent. It extends from the diaphragm above and continues as the pelvic cavity — containing the bladder and rectum (and uterus in the female) — below. Its bony limits are the ribs above and the pelvic bones below. Many of the upper abdominal organs such as the liver, stomach, spleen and kidneys lie partly covered by the lower ribs (see Figs. 34 and 35).

The abdominal muscles — the rectus abdominis and oblique muscles — protect the contents at the front and flanks. Behind is the vertebral column clothed with powerful vertebral muscles.

The abdomen moves as we breathe in and out. This outward movement on inspiration is most noticeable in men. Women tend to breathe using their chest muscles.

Contents of the abdomen

The diagrams demonstrate the approximate position of the intra-abdominal organs. The LIVER is the largest. It occupies the upper right portion but also extends over to the left of the upper abdomen. The STOMACH occupies the upper left side. Below these two organs the large and small bowel fill the cavity. Behind the stomach lies the PANCREAS (not illustrated). This digestive gland also produces insulin to keep the blood sugar level controlled. It is fish-shaped and lies across the vertebral column, against which it can easily be compressed and torn by a hard blow. Its digestive juices will then leak out, producing serious inflammation.

In the gutter formed by the lower ribs and the backbone lie the KIDNEYS. They are vulnerable to attack and injury from the roundhouse kicks, punches or poor breakfalls. On the left side the SPLEEN lies under the ribs. This is a most vulnerable

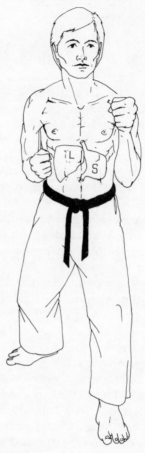

Fig. 34 The position of the upper abdominal organs (diagrammatic).
L = Liver   S = Stomach

organ. It bleeds easily and can be ruptured by kicks or punches.
INJURIES TO THE ABDOMINAL CONTENTS ARE
POTENTIALLY LIFE-THREATENING. The liver, spleen
and kidneys bleed profusely if seriously injured. The stomach
and pancreas, if ruptured, will cause serious inflammation of the
membrane inside.

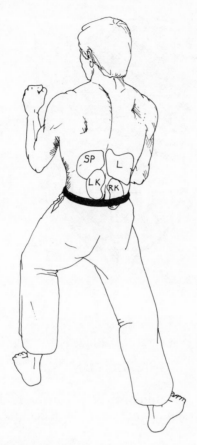

Fig. 35 The position of the upper abdominal organs (diagrammatic back view). L = Liver   Sp = Spleen   LK = Left Kidney   RK = Right Kidney

INJURIES TO THE SKIN

Abrasions, lacerations and bruises are all relatively common. Their treatment is along standard lines. One especially important type of abrasion is called 'patterned abrasions'. If after a crushing fall or hard blow an individual has abdominal pain and the impression of his belt or short elastic is deeply marked on the skin over the site of the blow, this may mean intra-abdominal injury. Observe the injured person closely. He may require to be taken to hospital.

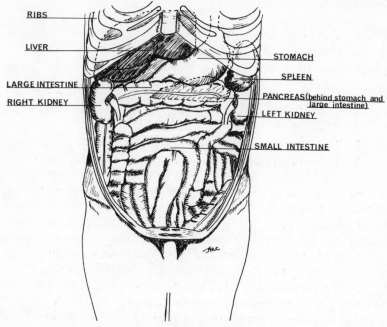

Fig. 36 The contents of the abdominal cavity.

INJURIES TO MUSCLE

Bruises of the abdominal muscles can be both extensive and painful. They respond well to the ICE regime.

INJURIES TO THE ABDOMINAL CONTENTS

Organs such as the liver, spleen and kidneys BLEED after injury. The stomach if burst *leaks acid*. The pancreas leaks *digestive juices* into the abdominal cavity. If the bowels are ruptured they will *leak liquid faeces* into the abdomen.

These produce specific signs and symptoms.

Symptoms

1. The person feels sweaty and clammy.
2. He complains of abdominal pain either over the whole abdomen or only over that part which was hit.
3. He may complain of shoulder-tip pain.

Signs

1. The person is clammy to the touch.
2. The pulse becomes faster, weaker and sometimes irregular.
3. Breathing is shallow and fast.
4. The abdomen is tender to touch and may be rigid due to involuntary muscle spasm. This rigidity does not relax with time.
5. The person may become progressively paler.
6. The temperature may rise and produce facial flushing if the cause is a ruptured pancreas, bowel or stomach.

The complaint of pain in the shoulder is caused by irritation of the diaphragm by blood or acid, etc. It is a misinterpretation by the brain and is due to stimulation of the phrenic nerve which supplies both the shoulder and the diaphragm.

Your action in the presence of these signs and symptoms is to arrange for hospital transfer by ambulance. While waiting, keep the injured person warm. Let him lie with his head to one side. Do not give any fluid by mouth and note his pulse rate at regular intervals — say every five minutes. Elevate his limbs on pillows.

More minor injuries may present with symptoms only after 12–24 hours. Blood in the urine on passing water may represent kidney damage. This should always be reported to your doctor. If there is very heavy bleeding then hospital attendance is recommended.

There are other rare examples of abdominal injuries which probably formed the basis of the mystical 'Ten day kill' or 'One year kill' described in ancient martial arts. Sometimes the liver or spleen gets damaged but seals itself after bleeding only a little. Usually about ten days later (rarely longer) this initial 'patch' is knocked off with straining or active exercise. Collapse can suddenly occur due to the bleeding which then follows. Your action should be the same as described above.

SERIOUS ABDOMINAL INJURY IS NOT COMMON. IT IS IMPORTANT THAT YOU HAVE KNOWLEDGE OF THE ABDOMINAL ORGANS FOR THIS WILL PERMIT EARLY RECOGNITION OF POTENTIAL CATASTROPHE.

17.
INJURIES TO THE ARM, WRIST AND HAND

ANATOMY OF THE ARM, WRIST AND HAND

The upper limb consists of the shoulder blade (scapula), the collar bone (clavicle), the bone of the arm (humerus), the forearm (radius and ulna), the wrist and the hand. They are covered with the muscles of the shoulder and arm. Extensions of the forearm muscles into tendons allow fine finger movements to take place.

Study Fig. 14. The muscles of the shoulder and shoulder blade allow almost complete rotation of the arm. The biceps muscle along with its neighbour — the brachialis — flexes the forearm. The triceps muscle straightens the elbow. It is the 'locking-out' muscle of weight-lifters. Its development in punchers gives sharpness to jabs and straight punches. In the forearm, flexion and extension of the wrist and fingers is performed by the muscle groups arising from the radius and ulna.

There are three important nerves in the arm. One of these is injured at the elbow and is colloquially called 'the funny bone'. This is the ULNAR NERVE. Injury produces tingling of the little and ring fingers of the hand. The RADIAL NERVE winds round the humerus and is especially liable to injury in the middle part of the upper arm. Weakness of the wrist and grip results. The third nerve is the MEDIAN NERVE. This is rarely injured in combat sports.

FACT: Injuries to the upper limb are amongst the most common in combat sports. Hand injuries are especially disabling, causing loss of training and working time.

INJURIES TO THE SKIN

Bruises are common and resultant upon defensive manoeuvres. The ICE regime is most effective.

INJURIES TO MUSCLE AND TENDON

The shoulder muscle can be strained or torn in punches or attempted throws. Pain is located over the front of the shoulder and is made worse by shoulder movement.

The biceps muscle occasionally sustaines rupture of its upper tendon. An ugly painful bump on the arm results. Although unsightly, it does not produce any functional problems, for the strength of the arm is more dependent on the brachialis muscle. The lower tendon of the biceps at the crook of the elbow may become inflamed from overuse. This will require rest and gradual rehabilitation.

Triceps can be torn or overused too. Overuse injury is more common. It is caused by punching without a target. This is common in traditional karate. There is pain at the elbow, especially when it is snapped straight.

Treatment

Strains and tears must be immediately treated with the ICE regime. Overuse injuries require rest, ice, possibly anti-inflammatory treatment and perhaps physiotherapy. Return to sport should aim to avoid recurrence of old problems. Punches should be directed against a target. Sometimes strapping is required.

Tennis elbow

Pain on the outside part of the elbow is called tennis elbow. It is usually accompanied by tenderness and discomfort on rotation of the forearm.

Rest is important. All movements which produce the pain must be stopped, as this condition is notorious for becoming a chronic problem. It is not a condition which you should treat yourself. If you have this problem you should contact your doctor for advice.

Golfer's elbow

This complaint affects the inside of the elbow and is produced by forcible stretching of the ligaments and muscles at this site.

Arm locks or twists are the most common causes.

Rest and ice are important. The problem is usually self limiting. Symptoms last up to six weeks.

INJURIES TO BONES AND JOINTS

The shoulder blade

The shoulder blade can be broken from a kick or during a fall. Marked swelling and tenderness are the rule. The diagnosis is confirmed by X-ray and most often no treatment is required because healing is rapid (two to three weeks).

Dislocation of the shoulder

This is the injury of wrestling or judo. The schoolboy trick of forcing the arm up the back tears the shoulder capsule and lets the joint dislocate forwards. The appearance is typical (Fig. 37).

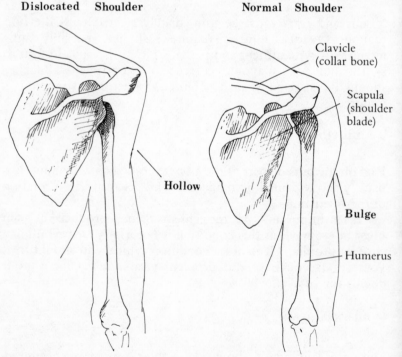

Fig. 37 How to recognise a dislocated shoulder.

The arm is held close to the body. There is severe pain and examination reveals an obvious step below the outer edge of the collar bone. Do not try heroically to put the joint back in place because a fracture might also be present. If it is, you could seriously damage blood vessels and nerves in the arm. Rather, place a rolled bandage or wad of gauze in the armpit and gently apply a broad sling or bandage the arm to the patient's body — whichever is most comfortable. Arrange for IMMEDIATE hospital transfer where the deformity will be confirmed and reduced.

Recurrent dislocation sometimes happens. If you have had a dislocated shoulder, do not take part in strenuous activity for six to eight weeks afterwards to allow the tissues time to heal.

Fractures of the humerus

These uncommon injuries can be hairline fractures only or displaced fractures which produce unsightly deformity. Pain is common to both types and medical advice is required. To increase the injured person's comfort during hospital transfer, place a pad in the armpit and bandage the injured limb to the side of the body as illustrated.

Such injuries take six to twelve weeks to heal depending on their severity. As soon as movements can be started, work within the limits of pain or stiffness to get the shoulder and elbow moving fully. These two joints do tend to stiffen when the upper arm is immobilised after a fracture. Full recovery can be expected within a month of removing the dressings.

Elbow injuries

The elbow joint is made up of the lower end of the humerus and the upper ends of the radius and ulna. In young people up to sixteen years old the bones have not yet fully developed and overuse injuries can occur quite easily. The cartilages of the growing bones can be pulled, producing pain and swelling.

The opinion of a doctor must be sought. Usually a training lay-off of from three to four weeks will be required until the symptoms settle.

Injury can also result from breaking objects with the point of the elbow. These can range from simple bruising to broken bones. Consideration should also be given as to whether it is

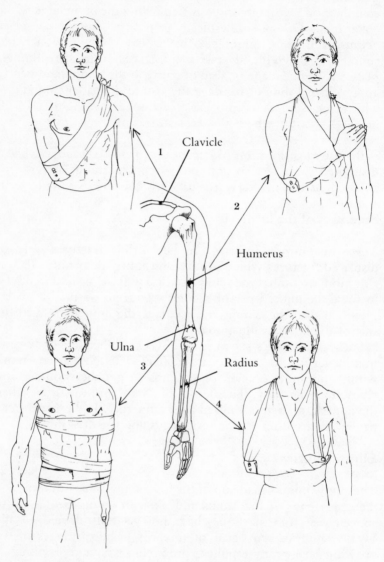

Fig. 38 Fractures of the upper limb. First Aid treatment.

really necessary to use the elbow in breaking techniques. Over a period of years joint changes can take place, eventually producing arthritis.

Treatment of all elbow injuries involves ICE in the immediate post-injury phase. More commonly a lay-off with anti-inflammation drugs such as aspirin or paracetamol is needed. Fractures require immobilisation in plaster. A stiff elbow may result from a fracture.

Fractures of the radius and ulna

The forearm bones are broken under the following situations:
1. Parrying blows, usually kicks.
2. Poorly executed breakfalls.
3. Twisting manoeuvres and falls onto the outstretched hand.

The recognition of such injuries is usually not very difficult. The person will complain of pain and will not be able to use the affected arm. You should have no hesitation in making the painful limb comfortable by placing it in a broad arm sling as illustrated in Fig. 38. Remember to give nothing by mouth and to take the injured person to hospital.

Injuries to the wrist

There are light small bones in the wrist. One of them, called the scaphoid, is frequently broken in falls on to the outstretched hand. This is an important injury for it can go unnoticed, being passed off as a sprain. This can lead to poor fracture healing and arthritis of the wrist in later life.

There is pain in the wrist with tenderness in certain positions, especially over the outside area of the wrist just below the root of the thumb. Often even the initial X-ray will show no break, but strapping of plaster of Paris is applied and the wrist re-X-rayed ten days to two weeks later. If a fracture is present it will show up on this occasion. Such an injury will lead to at least three months being lost.

Dislocations, fractures and sprains of the fingers

The knuckle bones of the striking fist are often injured in punching sports. Callosities over the index and middle finger knuckles act as protective pads in boxers and karatekae. On occasion they may become inflamed, or even develop deposits of calcium. They are then tender. Punching is impossible due to pain. Relief is best obtained by ICE and ASPIRIN or PARA-

CETAMOL.

The NECKS of the punching knuckles can be broken. The external appearance is shown in Fig. 39. Hospital treatment is required since deformity can produce disability if treatment is late or incomplete. Do not manage such problems yourself.

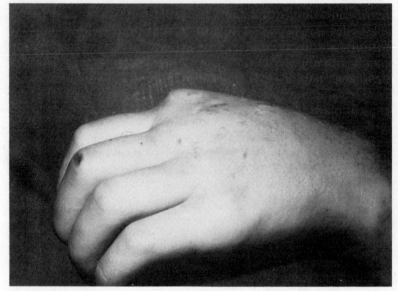

Fig. 39 Appearance of a broken knuckle bone.

The injured person will experience pain on punching up to three months afterwards. Rehabilitation therefore must be very gradual using adequate padding and strapping.

Another common fracture occurs at the BASE OF THE THUMB. This is illustrated with a fracture dislocation injury, for the two are very frequently encountered in boxers.

Specialist treatment in hospital is essential. The thumb is the most important digit. Its function should not be impaired by poor initial management.

Dislocations

Dislocations and sprains of the fingers have happened to most combat sportsmen/women. A dislocation is immediately apparent. The finger joints are out of line and the digit is numb. If seen immediately a firm pull holding the bones on each side of the joint will reduce the dislocation. Attempt this once only. If unsuccessful, the injury must be treated in hospital. Gently tape the injured finger to its neighbour to provide pain relief and splintage.

Sprains

Each little joint of the fingers is kept stable by ligaments. These can easily be sprained in combat. Immediately instigate the ICE regime if the pain is severe. No bandaging is necessary. The hand should be used as freely as possible afterwards.

After treatment of any hand injury the injured part should be elevated. This will mean sitting/lying with the hand and arm on a pillow so that the forearm and hand are above the heart. This allows the tissue fluid, which accumulates due to injury, to escape, thus preventing joint stiffness.

INJURIES TO NERVES

The radial nerve in the mid part of the upper arm and the ulnar nerve (funny bone) are the only two common injuries.

The radial nerve

This gives sensation to the skin on the back of the forearm and hand. It also supplies power to the strong extensor muscles of the arm and hand. Mawashi geri to the mid upper arm can injure this nerve. Immediately weakness in the wrist and grip is felt. It is impossible to make a tight fist. Numbness will be present to a varying extent over the back of the hand and forearm.

Historically this is an interesting nerve centre. It is said that if a swordsman was kicked strongly in the mid arm he would be unable to wield his weapon. Certainly the grip is weakened. If you grip something very tightly you will see that you must extend your wrist to do so. The ancient report is probably factual.

Treatment requires rest alone. The nerve is not severed but only bruised. Although tingling and weakness can last several weeks, recovery is usually complete. Remember though that if there is extreme pain a fracture may also be present and it will be necessary to attend the hospital casualty department.

The ulnar nerve

The 'funny-bone' lies just under the skin on the inside of the elbow. Injury produces an almost sickening tingling sensation of the little and ring fingers of the hand. Mostly a stray foot has caused the damage (and also sustained injury itself!)

Recovery is the norm and symptoms will disappear in minutes. If not, don't forget the possibility of a fracture, especially if the injury happened during breaking techniques. Visit the casualty department.

18.
INJURIES TO THE THIGH, LEG AND FOOT

ANATOMY OF THE THIGH, LEG AND FOOT

The lower limb consists of the buttocks, the thigh, the knee, the calf and the foot. Its bony support comes from the pelvic bones, the thigh bone (femur), the knee-cap, the tibia, the fibula (bones in the lower leg) and the bones of the foot. It has three main joints — THE HIP, THE KNEE and THE ANKLE — all of which are supported by large muscles, ligaments and tendons.

In combat sports, injuries can occur from two causes:
1. OVERUSE — roadrunning, kicking practice.
2. DIRECT VIOLENCE — e.g. from sweeps, kicks, twisting movements.

We shall deal with each area of the lower limb in turn, but special detail will be given to the regions most often injured.

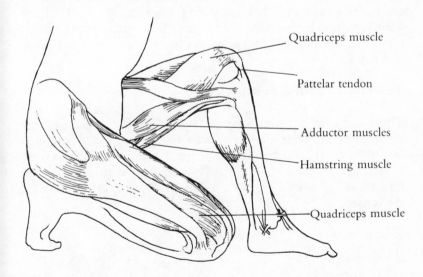

Fig. 40 Diagrammatic view of muscle of lower limbs. Notice the adductor muscle and the hamstring muscles inserting into the bones of the leg. These are the inner tendons which can be felt when the knee is bent.

Refer to the diagrams of the lower limb. Examine your own legs and try to identify the bones and muscles as we discuss them. Can you think of any injury situations affecting the lower limbs?

INJURIES TO THE PELVIS AND HIP

The pelvis consists of three bones, two pelvic bones and a part of the back formed by the backbone. It is called the SACRUM. Attached to the pelvic bones on each side is the hip joint. It is a ball and socket joint — very stable and rarely injured.

PROBLEMS

Clicking hip

Judoka and karateka who do a lot of stretching exercises sometimes develop clicking hips. As you go down with your legs apart you may hear a loud 'clunk', usually not painful. This is caused by a tight muscle band sliding over the outer part of the joint. Do not be worried about this. It is fairly common. If, however, it is painful, make an appointment to see your doctor and it will be investigated.

Tears of the adductor muscles

These are the muscles on the inside of the thigh. Over-enthusiastic stretching exercises can cause the muscle origin to be pulled off its attachment in the groin region of the pelvis — sometimes with a splinter of bone. This produces pain immediately, especially on stretching or whenever the muscles are tensed.

Treatment

If the injury occurs, ice pack the area AS SOON AS POSS-IBLE. After the initial pain has passed off, make an effort to use the muscles gently in stretching movements, but always within the limits of pain. Two soluble aspirin taken at the time of injury and four hourly afterwards for the first day will assist pain relief. Thereafter you should take aspirin three or four times per day for five to seven days.

Recurrent groin pain

Sometimes a fighter will present with an aching in the groin. It may be related to a specific injury episode or may have come on gradually. The pain may settle once he is warmed up, but ultimately he is unable to train. He should be referred to his doctor. Any overuse injury which does not settle quickly demands medical attention. The doctor, having carried out any necessary investigations, may then enlist the attention of a physiotherapist who can prescribe a specific treatment regime.

Avulsion fractures

Violent muscular activity in an adolescent or child athlete may avulse (tear away) a piece of bone or cartilage from the muscle or tendon's attachment. The muscles most often involved are the hamstrings and the rectus femoris muscle in the quadriceps.

Diagnosis

The injured area looks normal, but the site of the avulsion is tender. Any resisted movement produces pain at the site and the final diagnosis is confirmed by X-ray. You should therefore get a medical opinion.

Treatment will usually involve rest, analgesic drugs and gentle remobilisation after several days. Remember it is a fracture and will take time to heal completely.

INJURIES TO THE THIGH

The thigh muscles are the QUADRICEPS muscles at the front and the HAMSTRINGS at the back. They are attached to the pelvis above and the knee-cap (quadriceps) and tibia and fibula (hamstrings) below. Not surprisingly the most common injuries are to these muscles. The femur (thigh bone) is rarely injured in combat.

PROBLEMS

Bruising

A direct blow to the front of the thigh will produce varying degrees of bleeding within the skin and thigh muscle. There is sudden pain followed by a deep dull ache. Often obvious swelling develops. The pain is caused by pressure in the muscle due to bleeding.

Treatment consists of cold application and a compression bandage. Elevate the affected limb. In severe cases a day or two in bed may be necessary to let the swelling settle. DO NOT MASSAGE thigh injuries. We think this can produce complications and delay healing. In the few days after injury you should carefully limit all activity. By so doing one serious complication — that of bone forming in the muscle clot — can be avoided.

In very severe injuries HOSPITAL CONSULTATION in the first twenty-four hours may be required.

Muscle strains and ruptures

The quadriceps muscle is most often affected, the hamstrings less commonly. Following a direct blow there is severe pain, swelling and a 'dead leg' feeling. Gradually the pain settles but the leg remains stiff and weak. There is tenderness at the site of injury and sometimes a gap can be felt in the muscle. Any attempt to tense the muscle produces pain.

Treatment Cold application, compression and elevation remain the basis of effective first aid. Pressure should be applied for up to seventy-two hours. Subsequent treatment might involve the physiotherapist. Gentle exercises once the pain has settled maintain the muscle in its trained condition.

Sometimes adhesions and stiffness form some time later. If you have a persistent muscle injury, consult your club doctor. He will be able to advise you on how to improve performance.

Hamstring tears

These can be caused by direct injury or overstretching. Treat them as above.

The symptoms are of sudden pain in the back of the leg, the buttock crease, or the back of the knee. These are made worse by running or squatting.

Definitive treatment involves gentle exercises and gentle stretching. Physiotherapy help is often required.

INJURIES TO THE KNEE

The knee is a complex joint made up of the lower end of the thigh bone and upper end of the tibia. Sitting in front of the knee joint is the KNEE-CAP or PATELLA.

Take two chairs. Sit on one and place your heel on the other. Let your leg relax. Can you move your knee-cap from side to side? Now tighten your quadriceps (thigh muscles) on the front of your leg. You cannot move your knee-cap now because the quadriceps muscles steady the knee-cap when they are tense. A ligament runs from the lower part of the knee-cap into the tibia. It is called the PATELLAR TENDON.

The knee joint itself is made up of four ligaments and two cartilages. These are demonstrated diagrammatically in Fig. 41. All of these structures can be injured. Some produce minor aches. Others may require surgical treatment.

When a fighter has a knee injury ask yourself three questions:
1. Is the knee-cap broken?
2. Are the ligaments damaged?
3. Are the cartilages torn?

It will also be helpful to have knowledge of how the injury happened. So if you didn't see it yourself, ask the injured person or a spectator. You should ask:
1. Was there a blow to the knee directly or to the leg below?
2. Was the knee bent or straight?
3. Was the fighter's weight on his knee?

Now examine the joint and compare it to the uninjured side. Let the person keep his knee in the position that is most comfortable for him. Carefully look for any swelling. If it is present, and there is pain on feeling the knee or knee joint and the person is incapable of straightening his leg, he should be seen at hospital AS SOON AS POSSIBLE. Nothing is gained

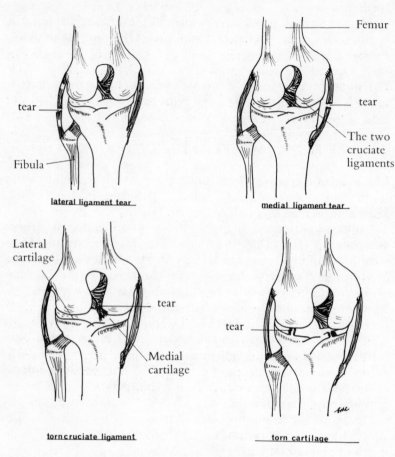

Fig. 41 Ligament and cartilage tears of the knee.

by continued cumbersome palpation of a painful knee. X-ray will confirm whether a fracture is present either in the knee joint itself or to the knee-cap.

TYPES OF INJURY

Injuries to the knee-cap

Bruising is the most common. It can be due to a slip when

boxing, a throw in judo or wrestling, or bumping one's knee on the ground after a karate sweep. There is usually obvious bruising or grazing and some pain on movement, but the leg can be straightened and tenderness is localised to the knee-cap itself. Apply the ICE regime. Let the fighter have a quick shower and apply a commercially-available knee bandage such as LASTONET (Lastonet Ltd.) or DOUBLASTIC (Boots Co.) This should stay on for forty-eight hours. After this movement should be encouraged and full activity will follow shortly afterwards.

Ligament injuries

The knee has four ligaments. Two are right inside the joint, two are situated on either side of the joint just under the skin. Twisting movements of the knee produce the injury while the weight is fully taken on the leg. Mistimed throws, sweeps and even the roundhouse kick can lead to ligament sprains and tears. In the roundhouse kick it is the non-kicking leg which twists. This can sometimes produce knee strain. Overstretching will occasionally produce pain in the ligaments on the inside of the joint.

Most injuries are minor, but the possibility of serious injury exists. In minor sprains there is tenderness on either the inside or the outside of the knee. In major injuries the knee will 'bend in the wrong direction'.

Moderate and minor sprains will present with pain over the affected ligament. Apply the ICE regime and follow this after thirty minutes or so with a firm bandage. If there is severe pain, seek medical attention AS SOON AS POSSIBLE. In some cases the doctor will wish to examine the injury after two to three days. This is to make certain that the injury is not more extensive than initially thought.

Rehabilitation will involve exercise in which increasingly rapid turning movements are made.

Torn cartilage?

The cartilages are two C-shaped wedges between the femoral and tibial surfaces of the knee joint. They are attached to the tibia. Their function is obscure but they are thought both to act as shock absorbers and to allow the even spreading of joint fluid. They have no ability to repair themselves. When torn, they can form a loose body in the joint or be split in such a way as to interfere with the joint's movements. The patient may complain of two problems:

1. His knee suddenly gives way.
2. His knee 'locks' or 'jams' and cannot be immediately straightened.

A cartilage usually tears when the leg is weight bearing, the foot is fixed and the body rotates around this. At the time of injury there may be swelling and pain which settles, but the knee becomes a persistent source of problems (1. and 2. above) afterwards.

The initial treatment for such injuries is ice, but a medical opinion is required.

Knee problems in children and youths

When the knee is still growing the sites of knee tendon insertion (into the knee-cap and upper end of shin bone) can become inflamed. The only treatment for this is REST after a medical opinion has been sought. Further exercise makes the problem worse. Symptoms usually settle over three to four weeks and exercise can be restarted when there is absolutely no tenderness over the sites of injury. These are OVERUSE injuries (see Chapter 9).

IT IS IMPERATIVE TO ENSURE CORRECT ASSESS-MENT OF A KNEE INJURY. IF A FIGHTER HAS A PAIN-FUL, SWOLLEN OR WEAK KNEE HE SHOULD BE TOLD TO SEEK A MEDICAL OPINION. HE SHOULD NOT BE ALLOWED TO CONTINUE TRAINING.

INJURIES TO THE LOWER LEG

The two bones are the tibia, which bears the body weight, and the fibula, a strut-like bone which provides origin for the three groups of lower leg muscles. In the calf these are the GASTRO-CNEMIUS and SOLEUS. They form a tendon which is inserted into the heel bone — the ACHILLES TENDON. These are the power muscles. They provide the propulsive force for actions like sprinting or jumping. In combat they allow the fighter to move quickly into attack or defence. At the front of the leg there is another group of muscles which pull the ankle upwards. Feel them tense and relax as you move your foot up and down. Yet another group lets us evert the foot (turn it outwards). Other movements such as inversion and rotation are due to combined muscle action.

An important nerve is situated just below the knee. A blow in this area will cause weakness of the foot and lower leg. This particular injury settles in hours to weeks. No treatment is necessary although there is often considerable discomfort.

PROBLEMS

Fractures of the bones, strains at bone-muscle junctions, muscle strains, bruises and inflammation of the Achilles tendon are among the common problems. One less common but potentially serious injury is described in detail on page 159 for its recognition is necessary if serious complications are to be avoided.

Fractures

Direct blows from kicks or rotational strains (as in throwing techniques) may produce fractures. Some may go unnoticed, or may be passed off as bruising, especially fractures of the fibula. However, the mechanism of injury may encourage suspicion and first-aid measures can then be applied. Remember too that some fractures of the tibia or fibula can be associated with damage to the ligaments of the knee or ankle. This must be borne in mind when examining a knee or ankle problem.

First-aid measures

Carefully and gently examine the injured limb. Compare it to the other leg. Is there bony tenderness? Is the individual incapable of standing on the leg? Feel both feet in fractures which are compound or have obvious deformity. Is there a temperature difference? If so, HOSPITAL ATTENDANCE is required immediately.

Splint the limbs. If your club has an inflatable splint, as it should have, remember to let it down slowly every half an hour and reinflate it if the journey to hospital is long.

Depending on the site and type of fracture, a period of from three to thirty weeks may be necessary before healing is complete! All advice given regarding training again must be understood and followed. There is no short cut to total rehabilitation.

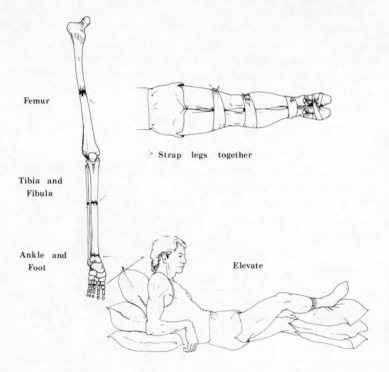

Fig. 42 Treatment of lower limb fractures.

Stress fractures

These are overuse injuries. The most well known occur in young soldiers who have been on forced marches. The repetitive striking of the foot on the ground leads to fracture of two foot bones. The injury heals with rest.

Sportsmen especially prone to this injury are footballers; they tend to suffer from stress fracture of the fibula. Ballet-dancers and long-distance runners can suffer from tibial or even vertebral fractures in the spine. Activities such as repetitive heavy roadwork are most liable to produce the injuries. If you suffer a chronic ache in the back or leg, think of this injury as a possibility. With rest of about four to six weeks the symptoms settle and gentle training should be restarted. A fracture requires rest to heal. This is one instance where you *must* stop training.

Fractures due to direct violence are uncommon in all combat sports in the tibia and fibula. However the lower ends of both bones can be broken in twisting movements of the lower leg on a fixed foot. This will result in the fracture illustrated. It is called a POTTS FRACTURE after the doctor who first described it.

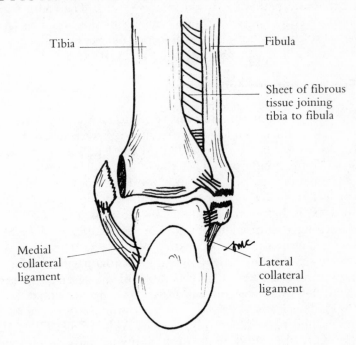

Fig. 43 Pott's fracture of the ankle.

There is usually a twisting injury, followed by marked ankle swelling and tenderness. The victim cannot weight-bear. The foot often feels dead. Look at the diagram. You will see that the fracture involves the bones around the ankle joint. To fix this correctly almost always requires surgery of some sort. If such an injury arises in your club, gently apply the inflatable splint or transport the patient with his foot placed on a supporting pillow and with the legs and feet gently bandaged together.

THIS INJURY REQUIRES HOSPITAL TREATMENT. IF YOU SUSPECT IT, DO NOT DELAY IN TRANSFER- RING THE INJURED PERSON TO HOSPITAL.

Shin splints

This is the name given to symptoms of pain in the front of the leg. Especially common amongst runners, it can occur whenever repetitive roadwork is involved. The cause may be stress fracture, muscle strain, bruising of the bones or lack of blood to the leg muscles. If the condition persists after rest and the ice regime, CONSULT A DOCTOR.

Tibial compartment syndrome

Our reason for mentioning this condition is that it is potentially very common in knock-down styles of karate where frequent sweeps or kicks may be landed on the leg. Running can also produce the condition.

The name applies to the muscles on the front of the leg. You can feel them tense if you pull your foot up strongly. These muscles lie between two bones — the tibia and fibula — and are strongly encased in tough fibrous tissue called FASCIA. This is an anatomical peculiarity of the leg. If there is severe bruising (with subsequent swelling) of this part of the leg, the muscle cannot swell visibly because of the fascia. But it does swell and by doing so compresses the artery which gives it blood. This leads to severe pain and numbness between the first and second toes. When this happens ALL ACTIVITY MUST BE STOPPED. Elevate the limb, apply ice and request medical attention. Serious consequences such as a local area of tissue death — GANGRENE — can result. This is a good reason for discouraging excessive low kicks and sweeps during bouts.

The condition may also occur in untrained road-runners. Therefore the motto is START SLOWLY and keep going until fitness improves. This will take at least four to six weeks. Then train harder. If symptoms occur, rest. Restart the schedule with shorter distances run over a longer period.

Achilles tendon injuries

The Achilles tendon is a potential weak spot in all athletes who do road-running. Its name derives from the mythical Greek hero Achilles, whose mother, Thetis, plunged him into the river Styx making his body invulnerable except for the heel by which she held him. He was killed after being wounded in the heel.

The commonest problems are:
1. Complete and partial rupture.
2. Achilles tendonitis and peritendonitis.

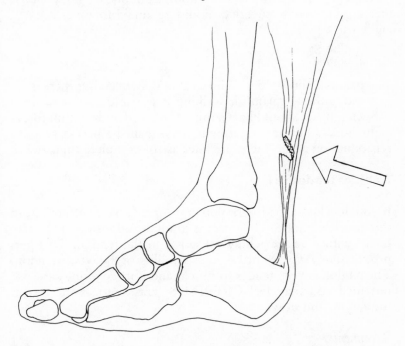

Fig. 44 Injury to the Achilles tendon. Complete or partial rupture can occur. More commonly the tendon and its coverings become inflamed.

Rupture

More commonly the older athlete suffers rupture but it can occur in young people, especially from a blow to the tendon. This has occurred recently in one young fighter in a crowded dojo.

Complete rupture

This is characterised by a snap or crack, with severe pain accompanied by inability to stand on tiptoe. On examination of the tendon you will see a defect. Feel it gently. There is a gap in the tendon.

Transport the person to hospital. He will require treatment in the form of surgery or plaster of Paris bandage. The injury can take six to twelve weeks to heal.

Rehabilitation Stretching exercises for the hamstrings and Achilles tendon should be practised within the limits of pain. Gradual increase in exercise severity should be aimed for over a six to eight week period.

Partial rupture

The pain is again sudden. The tendon is swollen but there is no gap and, although painful, walking is possible.

Such injuries should be examined by the doctor within forty-eight hours. Surgical treatment may again be necessary with rehabilitation along the same lines as for complete ruptures.

Achilles tendonitis

If you do a lot of roadwork you may already have suffered from this overuse injury. The onset is gradual and insidious. It may begin with a vague aching sensation in the tendon. This gets progressively worse until there is swelling of the whole tendon. The tendon is very tender to touch, and if its coverings are also inflamed you may feel CREPITUS (crackling) as the foot is moved up and down.

Treatment

Rest is an essential measure since efforts to 'run through' the condition will eventually lead to chronic tendonitis — a condition much more resistant to treatment. The period required is in the order of six weeks.

Heel raise The insertion of a heel raise of 1–2 cm inside the shoe can relieve symptoms considerably and even allow continued training.

Physiotherapy may be required in the form of ultrasound. Consult your doctor. He will prescribe physiotherapy if necessary.

Drugs Anti-inflammatory drugs are being increasingly used with encouraging results. Your doctor will decide whether these are necessary.

Surgery In spite of all these measures the symptoms may persist. On occasion surgery is necessary to relieve pain.

Rehabilitation

Avoid excessive strain on the tendon. Run on grass — not tarmacadam. Wear a heel raise and avoid strenuous uphill runs. Make sure too that your running shoes are of good quality with good support for the arch of your foot.

INJURIES TO THE ANKLE

About one fifth of all injuries in sport will occur to the ankle. It is in fact the most commonly injured joint in the body. The commonest injury is one of 'inversion' — that means the injury occurs by 'going over' on the joint with inward twisting of the foot. Such an injury usually happens suddenly and is characterised by pain and rapid swelling. The person can almost always bear weight if a sprain has occurred. This is not so if the bones are fractured. Injury most often occurs during roadwork or gym-training.

Anatomy of the ankle joint

Study the illustration of the ankle joint and the mechanism of injury. The ankle is a MORTICE joint made up of the lower ends of the tibia, fibula and their connection ligaments above and the talus bone of the foot below. The joint is supported on each side by strong ligaments and tendons. The talus acts as a ball-bearing in the mortice making the ankle a modified hinge joint.

Immediately after the accident the patient is often able to walk without discomfort, but within minutes the ankle begins to swell, becoming very painful.

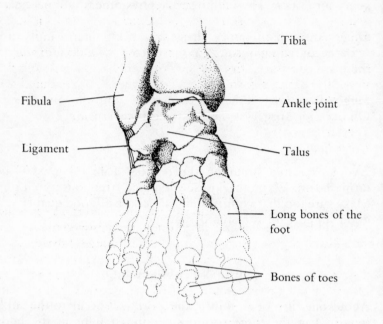

Fig. 45 The bones of the right ankle joint. Notice how the end of the fibula extends lower than the end of the tibia.

The aim of treatment is to support the ligament injury but enable walking with minimal discomfort. If there is extreme pain on weight-bearing or severe swelling, the patient should be seen early by the doctor.

Types of injury

Sprains of the ankle ligaments or fracture of the bones are injuries which frequently occur. It is vital that you differentiate between the two. Therefore assessment of each injury is essential.

At the time of injury it is possible to examine the ankle before it becomes swollen. This is ideal for it allows comparative inspection of the injured ankle and its normal neighbour. Very gently feel the bones around the joint. Are they very tender? Now feel below the lower ends of the ankle bones. This is where the ligaments lie. Is there tenderness here? Does it hurt to move the ankle?

Encourage the injured person to move his ankle through all normal movements, first on the floor, then supported and then alone. If he cannot do this, medical advice should be sought AS SOON AS POSSIBLE.

Treatment for sprains

Lateral ligament sprains are commonest and due to inward twisting of the foot. The usual routine of ice compression and elevation should be applied. Some form of supportive strapping should then be applied for up to forty-eight hours, after which it should be removed and the injured area reinspected. At this time there will be evidence of bruising or fullness of the hollows at the back of the joint. Encourage movements again at this stage to assess any discomfort. Now reapply strapping and adopt an active rehabilitation programme which initially involves movements of the joint only, gradually going on to weight-bearing and rotation exercises. Progress must be graded to avoid reinjury. Expect a period of up to four weeks for recovery. If injury recurs or does not settle, particular physiotherapy may be required.

19.
STRAPPING FOR INJURIES

Strapping satisfies two objects:
1. It provides physical support for the injured part, limiting pain but allowing mobility and rehabilitation. Thus the injured fighter can continue to train or compete.
2. It gives psychological support because if the injured part feels comfortable and stable there is no anxiety about using it.

We advise you to use strapping especially following ankle and knee injuries. It can also be effectively applied in finger and wrist injuries. It should only be applied once you have satisfied yourself that there is neither a fracture nor gross instability of the injured part. Apply it firmly but not so tightly as to cause discomfort. Remember that its function is to support injured ligaments and prevent painful movements. It should be applied after the initial injury has been inspected and basic first-aid treatment principles such as ICE completed.

The most valuable strapping materials are adhesive bandages (ELASTOPLAST, Smith and Nephew Ltd.). Supportive bandages (crepe) should be used in the treatment of fractures and dislocations. The following examples contain step-by-step instructions for application of strapping in the more common injuries. With practice you can become efficient in the techniques and be able to cope with 'niggling' injuries.

STRAPPING TECHNIQUES

Hand and wrist

Sprained wrist

Refer to Chapter 17 on arm, wrist and hand injuries. Remember that the diagnosis between sprain and fracture can often be extremely difficult. In doubtful injuries get a medical opinion.

An elastic bandage applied in the figure-of-eight style will give adequate support.

Method A 5 cm or 7.5 cm Elastoplast bandage should be used, depending on the size of the hand. The end should be cut for four or five inches to leave two tails, one broader than the other. These are laid, the narrow tail uppermost, across the palm. The bandage is then applied round the hand, split to support the thumb, and continued around the hand and wrist until sufficient support is given. Continue bandaging around the front of the wrist, across the back of the hand and over the palm in a figure of eight, splitting it to accommodate the thumb. The sequence should be repeated four or five times.

Thumb strapping

The figure-of-eight bandage is again aplied. This time use a 2.5 cm wide bandage.

Method Start just below the thumb joint. Apply two turns around the thumb (clockwise — right thumb, anticlockwise — left thumb). Then take the bandage across the palm, round the back of the hand and over the thumb. Now continue round the thumb and back across the palm. The process should be repeated for three or four turns, overlapping each turn and working down the palm and wrist.

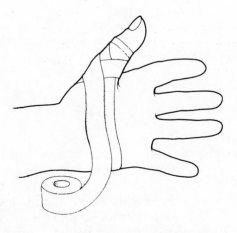

Fig. 46 How to strap a thumb strain

Finger injuries

Strap the injured finger to its neighbour by two lengths of
Elastoplast strapping. This method allows flexion of the fingers
but prevents sideways movement.

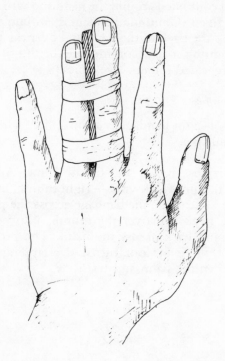

Fig. 47 How to strap a broken finger

Knee injuries

Minor strains and sprains should be strapped using 7.5 cm
bandages.

Method The knee should be slightly flexed and the foot resting
on a stool or chair. Use a safety razor to shave the hair around
the knee. Place a pad (either gamgee or cotton wool) behind the
knee and apply two Elastoplast strips of about 25 cm each as
illustrated around each side of the knee. Then apply bandaging

above and below the knee. The final turns should cover the knee itself.

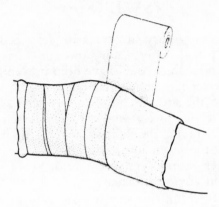

Fig. 48 How to strap a knee

Ankle injuries

You will recall that ankle injuries occur most often to the lateral ligaments. Strapping is therefore used to support this area.

Method A 7.5 cm wide bandage should be used. A single 'strap' should be applied after shaving the leg. One end should be applied to the inner calf and the other end extended to the outer calf. It should pass under the heel and be tense enough to gently evert the ankle. Then apply the bandage around the foot from outside inwards in order to pull the foot outwards. This circular bandage should finish just below the knee.

Strapping is an effective method in strains and sprains. It is essential that there is no doubt about the diagnosis. If you are uncertain, consult the club doctor.

20.
TWENTY QUESTIONS — ANY ANSWERS?

In this chapter twenty injury situations are described. Most of them actually happened. After reading this book, have you any suggestions as to how they could have been prevented?

1. An amateur boxer is sparring without a mouth-shield. He receives a blow to the mouth and loses two teeth. Six weeks later he presents to his doctor with a chronic discharge from his lower lip. On X-raying the soft tissues in his lips it is noticed that a fragment of tooth remains buried and has caused a chronic infection. There are several points worthy of comment. What action would you have taken:
   i)   To prevent the injury?
   ii)   To manage it once it has occurred?

2. A boxer is taking punishment badly. He is knocked down with hard punches to the head three times in one round and only just manages to get back to his feet each time before he is counted out. He receives a further combination of punches to the head and is knocked out. He recovers consciousness after twenty minutes.
   i)   Should he have been allowed to continue after three knock-downs or before three knock-downs occurred?
   ii)   When should he fight again?
   iii) Is it justifiable to avoid his being knocked out?

3. At a world championship in karate, officials are instructed to remove gum-shields from all competitors. Any comments?

4. A one-eyed individual takes part in free sparring at a karate lesson and is kicked in his good eye. When X-rayed he is found to have a blow-out fracture of the eye socket. He is now partially-sighted in that eye. How could this have been avoided?

5. A traditional fighter receives a combination of blows to the head and abdomen. He falls backwards to strike his head on the stone floor where the fight is taking place. He fractures his skull and needs neurosurgical treatment. Would you have anticipated this disaster?

6. At a full-contact competition the doctor approaches you as organiser of the event to say that he is unhappy about both the fitness and lack of a medical record of one of the fighters. You

are pushed for fights since one has already been called off.
What do you say to the doctor?

7. After a short period of post-traumatic amnesia from a minor
head injury, a fighter who refused to go to hospital because he
wanted to watch the rest of the competition becomes drowsy
when he returns home that evening. His wife smells alcohol on
his breath and supposes that he has had too much to drink.
However she cannot rouse him and sends for an ambulance. He
requires a neurosurgical operation to remove a clot of blood
from his brain and remains partially disabled.

   i)   Should his refusal to be seen at hospital be accepted?
   ii)   Is it wise to go drinking after a head injury?
   iii) Can you work out the sequence of events from the head
       injury to the drowsiness and subsequent coma?

8. A boxer, normally an average puncher, suddenly becomes a
knock-out specialist.

   i)   Would you accept this at face value and congratulate
       him?
   ii)   What are the possibilities other than the acquisition of
       good technique which could genuinely explain his new-
       found skills?

9. A woman begins karate lessons. At her second lesson she is
sparring and sustains several punches and kicks to her upper
abdomen. She feels very bruised but recovers, only to collapse
suddenly six weeks later. On this occasion an emergency
operation saves her life. Surgeons remove a large blood clot
from her liver (liver injury can produce symptoms long after
the initial blow).
Can you think of any way in which this situation could have
been prevented?

10. After a heavy throw on to his left side a judoka complains
that he has pain both in his upper abodmen and in his left
shoulder. He is clammy but says he will be all right.

   i)   What course of action will you take?
   ii)   What are the judoka's possible injuries?
   iii) What questions will you ask to confirm your suspicions?

11. After performing a souplesse technique, a young wrestler
complains of occasional numbness and tingling in the fingers of
his right hand.

   i)   What are his possible injuries?
   ii)   What action should you take?

12. At a kendo demonstration the shinai splinters and passes

through the face guard of the teacher. He sustains a fatal injury when the splinter passes into his brain by way of the eye socket. What would seem to be the main safeguard in preventing this type of tragedy?

13. At a karate lesson free sparring is taking place. One participant steps backwards and collides with one of the participants behind him. In a freak accident the man behind sustains a complete rupture of his Achilles tendon which requires surgical correction.
What methods would have prevented this 'accident'?

14. A fighter comes to you, his coach, to report a pulled muscle in his shoulder.
Do you tell him to fight on, saying it will go away?
If not, what first-aid treatment would you give?

15. When sparring with his instructor a karateka sustains the following injuries:
   a) Black left eye.
   b) Cut right eye.
   c) Broken front tooth.
These were the result of three separate collisions.
If you were involved in the running of the Sports Centre which permitted the karate classes to take place, what steps would you take to prevent this happening?
Is it possible that these injuries constitute assault?

16. As a female martial artist you sustain a punch to your right breast. After the bruising and pain settles down there is still a discrete, hard lump in your breast.
Would you ignore this and attribute it solely to the injury?
Would you consult your doctor?

17. You are attacked one night in the street from behind but because of your martial arts training you respond immediately and throw your attacker over your shoulders. He is temporarily dazed and you wait until he recovers with the intention of taking him to the police. However, you are so annoyed and upset that you begin to kick and punch him although he offers no resistance. Eventually the police arrive and both of you are detained. Witnesses at the scene have missed your initial defence manoeuvre.
Do you think that your punching the attacker could constitute self-defence? Could you be charged with assault?

18. A partially-sighted person wishes to train at your karate club. In allowing him to participate, what measures would you

take to safeguard his sight and thereby to prevent potential litigation against you should an accident occur?

19. The parents of a ten-year-old boy are anxious that their son becomes expert in judo because he is more studious than physically aggressive in school. Can you recognise any potential problems with such a student and his promoters?

What would you say to his parents regarding his lack of physical aggression?

Would you organise his training any differently from normal?

20. Do you feel, having read of these situations, that there is a need to improve general knowledge of injuries in combat?

Are the media overstating the problems?

Would increased awareness and first-aid training help the situation?

APPENDIX

MEDICAL RECOMMENDATIONS FOR REDUCTION OF INJURIES IN COMBAT SPORT

1. A medical certificate of fitness to compete should be presented before a contest.
2. Each fighter should carry a fight record card on which is recorded previous performances and injuries.
3. A doctor should be present at competitions.
4. Following an injury to the eye, ear or head the competitor must be re-examined medically before fighting again. A minimum of four weeks should elapse before fighting again after a head injury (knock-out).
5. Equivalent weight classes are encouraged. Ideally, no fighter should outweigh his opponent by more than seven pounds (7 lb).
6. Referees and instructors should be encouraged to learn first aid.
7. The governing body should issue a summary of the rules of the sport. They should be freely available to all members of the association.
8. Before competitions a summary of the rules should be announced.
9. Suitable protective equipment must be worn and specifically recommended by the governing body in liaison with the medical officer to the sport.
10. Dangerous manoeuvres should be banned.
11. During training and warm-up, adequate space and lighting is necessary.
12. Sprung or matted flooring is recommended.
13. Get yourself insured against injury under a recognized Combat Sports scheme. For oriental arts the Martial Arts Commission (15–16 Deptford Broadway, London SE8 4PA, Tel: 01 691 3433) will help.
14. Join only Sports-Council-recognized clubs.

INDEX